Who Owns Our Bodies?

making moral choices

D0771967

DATE DUE

Who Owns Our Bodies?

making moral choices in health care

JOHN SPIERS

Health Policy Adviser
The Social Market Foundation

Visiting Fellow, The King's Fund Management College

Chairman, The Patients Association

Radcliffe Medical Press
Oxford and New York

in association with the
Institute for Health Policy Studies,
University of Southampton

I|H|P|S

Radcliffe Medical Press Ltd
18 Marcham Road, Abingdon, Oxon OX14 1AA, UK

Radcliffe Medical Press, Inc.
141 Fifth Avenue, New York, NY 10010, USA

British Library Cataloguing in Publication Data

A catalogue record for this book is available from the British Library.

ISBN 1 85775 210 4

Library of Congress Cataloging-in-Publication Data is available.

Typeset by Advance Typesetting Ltd, Oxon
Printed and bound in Great Britain by
Biddles Ltd, Guildford and King's Lynn

'Before you begin building these great systems, let us make sure what the bricks are made of.'

GE Moore

'The ultimate goal of life is life itself.'

Alexander Herzen

'Just mix up a mixture of theolologicophilolological. *Mingo, minxi, mictum, mingere.*'

James Joyce

'... here is the strangest controversy
Come from the country to be judged by you.'

King John

'O me, the word "choose"!'

The Merchant of Venice

'But that the dread of something after death,
The undiscovered country, from whose bourn
No traveller returns, puzzles the will,
And makes us rather bear those ills we have
Than fly to others that we know not of?'

Hamlet

Dedication

For Leigh, naturally

The author

John Spiers is Chairman of The Patients Association, a national charity campaigning for patients' rights. John is also Health Policy Adviser to the Social Market Foundation, the leading policy 'think tank', and a consultant on health care management. He has had two successful careers: firstly, as the founder of four book publishing companies, and a winner of The Queen's Award for Export Achievement in 1986, and secondly as a policy adviser on health and education.

His book, *The Invisible Hospital and the Secret Garden: an insider's commentary on the NHS reforms*, is published jointly by Radcliffe Medical Press and the Institute of Health Services Management. He is also the author of a major study of empowerment, in *Sense and Sensibility in Health Care* (edited by Marshall Marinker) published by BMJ Publishing in 1996, and of the forthcoming guide, *How to be a Streetwise Patient*.

He has been Chairman of Brighton Health Authority, Brighton Health Care NHS Trust and the South East Thames RHA Salomons Centre, for management development. He is a Visiting Fellow of the NHS Staff College – Wales and of the King's Fund Management College.

He also has extensive Whitehall experience, having been an advisor to the Prime Minister on the Citizens' and the Patients' Charter and a member of the NHS Executive and ministerial advisory groups on corporate governance, openness in the NHS, communications, and the Patients' Charter. He now serves on the NHS Executive Patient Responsiveness Working Group and is also a ministerial advisor on design and patient care.

John appointed the first ever Patients' Advocate inside an NHS provider Trust, and established the first Clinical Performance Improvement Unit in the NHS.

His other interests are in the arts and education. He is Chairman of the educational charity The Trident Trust, Vice-Chairman of the Grant Maintained Schools Foundation, and a member of the Court of the University of Sussex, which awarded him an honorary doctorate in 1994.

Contents

Foreword

Medicine is a complex area in which uncertainty and lack of information are endemic. This state of affairs provides the overriding rationale for an agency relationship; that is, an arrangement whereby patients rely upon better-informed professionals to act as their agents in many areas of decision–making. However, the necessity for this dependence raises many problems of its own. How does the patient judge the expertise of the agent? How can the agent know the patient's preferences, wants and needs? How can we be sure that the agent acts in the patient's interests? These are just some of the pressing questions that arise. It is also the world that John Spiers addresses in this thoughtful and challenging book *Who Owns Our Bodies?*

John Spiers is a rare individual. He has a passion for ideas. He succeeds in combining unusually high levels of thought and action. Moreover, he is not afraid to address controversial issues. It was these qualities that prompted me to invite him to deliver a public lecture at the Institute for Health Policy Studies, University of Southampton. We were not disappointed. The broad and eclectic canvas upon which he presented his thoughts on the fundamental issues of patient choice, who decides about the quality of a life and user empowerment are set out in this book. His ability to draw on the works of eminent literary and philosophical thinkers in addressing practical modern day health dilemmas – an ability that gives his writing a distinctive quality – is amply demonstrated in the following pages. What cannot be demonstrated, however, is his willingness and ability to engage with questioners and critics in constructive debate about his ideas. There will always be those who disagree with him. But those who welcome a free market in ideas will value this latest contribution to health policy debate.

Professor Ray Robinson
Director, Institute for Health Policy Studies
University of Southampton
November 1996

A note on the text

This short book is an expansion of the public lecture I delivered on 16 April 1996, to the Institute for Health Policy Studies at the University of Southampton at the invitation of its director, Professor Ray Robinson. I am grateful to him for the opportunity to explore these ideas and for our discussions.

I am especially indebted, too, to Leigh Richardson for carefully reading and commenting valuably on a sequence of drafts, and to my friends John Simmonds and Bill Pickering for our unfinished conversations. The views expressed are, of course, my own. They are not necessarily shared by any of those organizations with which I am associated.

For publication, I have enlarged my discussion of Sir Isaiah Berlin's ideas and of three topics: the Tony Bland case, the so-called 'persistent vegetative state' (which I propose should be known instead as 'impaired capacity syndrome', since none of us is a thing) and the Australian discussions concerning *The Rights of the Terminally Ill Act 1995 (Northern Territory)* and voluntary euthanasia.

I have added an *Introduction*, written after the lecture was delivered. This has enabled me to set out in more detail the principles outlined then. As a result, I have transferred some of the initial conceptual paragraphs of my lecture to the *Introduction*. Otherwise, my lecture framework remains, although it supports a substantially extended text.

I have also added an *Afterword*, which takes account of some more recent cases, and which offers some further thoughts in these continuing and most delicate debates.

I am, as ever, indebted to Gillian Nineham, Editorial Director of Radcliffe Medical Press, for her continued encouragement of my work, and to Jamie Etherington, Editorial Manager, for his adroit editorial support and valued guidance.

My most fundamental debt is to the dedicatee of what is intended as a modest enquiry into a most difficult and challenging area of health care, where we reflect uncomfortably on who and what we are.

In writing this work I have been conscious of the Greek motto which Laurence Sterne displays on the title-page of the first volume of *Tristram Shandy*: 'It is not things themselves, but opinions concerning things, which disturb men.'

However, let's hold on to a comment from Thomas Eidson, in his novel *The Last Ride*: 'you weren't born in the woods to be scared by an owl.'

John Spiers
Old Portsmouth
November 1996

Introduction

Foundations

Shakespeare tells us that we do not need Banquo or the ghost in *Hamlet*, returned from the grave, to remind us that life and death are the most enigmatic, uniquely puzzling and formidable of subjects. Apparitions are not needed to stir belief and choice, autonomy and governance. For life's mystery, sanctity and dignity, its brevity and its context of universal infinity, all fix these enigmas to our view.

Who Owns Our Bodies? steps carefully in the land of *Hamlet*. It seeks to identify the key moral questions. It explores what is essentially a debate about what it is to be a human being.[1] The crucial questions are two: what is a person, and who should make choices for the individual? John Locke offered the definition of a person most commonly found.[2] He emphasized rationality and self-consciousness:

> A thinking intelligent being that has reason and reflection and can consider itself as itself, the same thinking being, in different times and places.

However, we have to consider the consequences of the different answers that people give in a world where traditional ethical guidance is foundering.

I explore these two themes and respond to these quandaries. First, I argue that we should relish the sanctity of life, and the civilized role of medicine in enabling the individual to be born, live and die as well as possible. Second, that we should emphasize self-realization and not coercion by government in these life and death choices. We should be, like James Joyce in his work, our own 'continuous copy'. For, as Ronald Dworkin, the University of Oxford's Professor of Jurisprudence, puts it:

> the underlying question is a more universal issue of political morality. Should any political community make intrinsic values a matter of collective decision rather than individual choice?[3]

The essential question is: what is it to be a human being? This is to ask when does a human creature acquire rights and interests, and what are these. Laurence Sterne declares in *Tristram Shandy*: 'I begin with writing the first sentence – and trusting to Almighty God for the second'.[4] His own famous initial lines said:

> I wish either my father or my mother, or indeed both of them, as they were in duty both equally bound to it, had minded what they were about when they begot me; had they duly considered how much depended upon what they were then doing.

It was then held, as he implies, that the moment of conception affected the embryo. Indeed, in the 18th century the spermatozoon was thought of as a miniature and perfect human being. We are less male-centric, but where does *our* first late-20th century sentence begin?

We are offered both absolute and relative answers as to who are the members of the moral community, and how their interests are to be protected. These answers are offered in response to the issues that arise when we consider what is a person and what is the moral basis of choice to be. Thus, we find these ethical entanglements: at what point does a human begin to embody both intrinsic and sacred value? When does human potential become determined? And what do we mean by species-membership? Is this, for example, extended to every sperm and egg? Or to every fetus, even if clearly so damaged as to be hardly recognizably human? Should a fetus be aborted for purely social reasons? Should fetuses be aborted when virtually capable of independent life? Should medicine be permitted to develop human embryos for research, and then be killed? Can fetal tissue transplantation be morally insulated from induced abortion? Is the unborn fetus a member of the moral community, and from which point?[5] Is this membership conditional, and if so, how and why? Does membership arise at conception and when is that? Or at birth? Or only if the child has certain agreed and given characteristics?

These knotty, and often labyrinthine, challenges turn on the ethical question as to whether or not there are limits to the means to life, and whether all available techniques should always be used to maintain life? Thus, are there *absolute* 'rights' (moral or legal) to life (or to death), or are these *relative* to responsibilities, to obligations (and to resources), which depend on circumstances? And if this latter is the case, what are the minimum requirements for a right to life, and how should these be determined? The same problems arise at the end of life, too, as will appear.

Here, we particularly confront two questions. First, of whether life must be preserved irrespective of its quality. And, second, that the acceptance and expression of the human, cultural, medical, and even spiritual response sets the expectations of the community. These ethical expressions establish our care conventions, our routines, and the approaches of professionals to their caring responsibilities (which should focus on 'benefit', which patients define). These moral expressions establish in the minds of patients those roles they are expected to assume.[6] The question of whether life must be preserved irrespective of its quality arises with the elderly, with the demented, with those in coma, and in considering how to act with the severely damaged infant. When we consider the beginning of life, definitions of life itself are problematic. When we consider the end of life, even the obvious is elusive. We continue to work with literary images, of 'the awful boundary between life and death', of 'the first of these sorrows which are sent to wean us from the earth'.[7] Yet what do we mean by death – Parson Yorick's empty black pages in *Tristram Shandy*. How do we know death has occurred? When does a human being die? When should medicine stop trying to prevent this, if ever? We think we know, in common sense. But ethicists offer uncommon answers.

Such questions have baffled many. Yet we do need guidance and a framework of legitimacy for daily, practical decision-making. Professionals, too, need to define their ethical position and act upon it before they face individual difficulties in individual cases of clinical practice. This suggests that society needs to set clear rules, which are themselves responsive to social changes. This does not imply the abandonment of the disabled and the disadvantaged. Indeed, the contrary is the case. However, a subjective and individual professional opinion is not necessarily a satisfactory basis for ethics. This is not to say that if the law establishes a framework for ethical decisions this should not set the individual free to make choices. Indeed, that is what is wanted, if we mean by the individual the recipient of the 'care'.

We each work with a concept of what it is to be human, however intuitive and un-argued this may be. Ethics and moral philosophy seeks to help us. A key concept offered is that of 'species-membership'. This is said to have both a secular and a spiritual basis. Yet difficulties arise in medical and social practice when we ask at what point (if at all) a human being commences or ceases to embody intrinsic and sacred value. This is to ask, with Sterne, some of those medical-cum-theological questions which he addresses, when he teases his readers by asking whether or not a child can be baptized before it is born. A great deal turns on how we think about these questions of moral community. For example, do we enter the moral community when we are first thought of? At or after conception? At or after birth? Do we leave the moral community when in a coma? Or when diagnosed as in a persistent vegetative state? Or when dementia develops? What is our moral status when born handicapped, or diagnozed as handicapped while still in the mother's womb? These are not what Sterne calls hobby-horse questions. For the answers we give define society. There are important personal and public policy consequences implied in how we answer what Shakespeare calls 'the music of men's lives.'[8]

We are asking about the most fundamental of fundamentals. These are more elusive than we expect them to be. The law, clearly, must define and revise. It must regulate change, discipline practice, assess and intrude upon motive and manner of action. The law is, too, intertwined both with achieving and reflecting social consent.

The most basic question is where should the line be drawn between coercion and self-discipline, between control and choice, between central action and personal autonomy? It is common ground between opposing parties and philosophies that we need, a much more satisfactory legal and ethical framework for soundly based choices concerning what it means to bring into being, prolong or end life. We need to sort out when, how, and on what grounds a human life has a claim to protection, and from whom – including from ourselves.

Two special claims are made about the notion of the sanctity of life. First, that there is special value in the life of a member of the human race. Second, that there is special value in the individual life of a person. The sanctity of human life is widely held to be of some special value. This is traditionally viewed as distinct from the value of the lives of other living things – for example, the lives of the higher apes closest to us in the evolutionary and DNA chain.[9] Indeed, this idea has been thought to have the most special status, that of divine sanction. It derives from the Hebrew view of creation, accounted in Genesis.[10] Thus the human situation in the divine plan:

> And God said, Let us make man in our image, after our likeness: and let them have dominion over the fish of the sea, and over the fowl of the air, and over the earth, and over every creeping thing that creepeth upon the earth ... and God said ... Be fruitful, and multiply, and replenish the earth, and subdue it; and have dominion over the fish of the sea and over the fowl of the air, and over every living thing that moveth upon the earth.

Some ethicists, notably Peter Singer, question the moral adequacy of this account. Singer queries what we mean by species-membership. He questions the justifications offered for the distinctions we use to isolate ourselves from the higher animals.[11]

These are ethical, constitutional and practical questions. They are predicaments for the individual and for the citizen. For this is not merely an abstract enquiry about who has morally relevant interests, and who has rights that protect those interests. These questions of sanctity, of membership in the moral community, of where boundaries properly lie are clearly identified and exemplified if we look at the challenges of both involuntary and voluntary euthanasia. Bleakly put, we ask how can any of us ever be better off dead? I am reminded of the extraordinary imagery and power of Bergman's film *The Seventh Seal,* which relies on the notion that we all play chess with death as we seek meaning in our lives. We each play chess in hope. We seek, in Samuel Beckett's terms, neither to despair nor to presume. Dworkin asks us to consider how might death itself give meaning to life, and be a completion, a rounding-out of life. We might ask, thus, how death itself can be both controlled and positive in its experience. How might death itself provide a foothold, instead of being a dark coast sliding by? Is there a way, in Paul Carter's words, for 'The story to be told ... replaced by the act of telling'?[12] I will argue that we should ethically seek to achieve a coherence between life and death. That we should seek an integrity which unites both life and death. Thus, the one can structure and celebrate the other. Thus, life and death may overlap each other and envelop each other, creating a narrative unit. This is the notion of the role of the artistic, even the creative element in how one might intrude one's whole self upon one's own inevitable death by seeking to control its nature, 'content' and timing. There could thus be an artistic as well as a moral content, which is not to suggest a sacrilegious formulation of such a necessarily final event.

The historian John Vincent, considering how to assess voting opinion in the past, speaks of Victorian poll books as 'door to door interviews with the dead'.[13] There is a crucial sense in which we need an interview, a re-definition *with the living*, with ourselves. We need what WB Yeats said characterized the novelist George Moore, 'the terrible gift of intimacy'. Life and death might be seen in William Empson's terms, as 'Two mirrors with Infinity to dine'.[14] We do need, like a third Irishman, Sterne himself, to enter fully the world we have ourselves created. This is to see death as critical to the achievement of our selves in living our lives, as is the life we *have* lived. It thus matters very much how each event of birth and death occurs, and how these inter-relate. Thus, death can be a 'working through' of the historical experience of one's own self-realization, a means to constitute the totality of experience, to give a life ethical and narrative meaning. Death can offer an expectation that it need not necessarily disrupt the entire meaning of a life, but complete it. Death need not falsify the life lived.

None doubt that death is itself both a linguistic and a human puzzle. We go only once, yet it is not even a first journey. No road exists. It is no journey at all. *The Tempest* tells us that we are 'such stuff as dreams are made of'. And yet, even despite Hamlet's musing, in that sleep of death no dreams may come. What then do we do if we choose it, plead for it, or impose it on another? Logic is not always a comfort.[15] For example, Singer says:

> being killed does not make us worse off; it makes us cease to exist. Once we have ceased to exist, we shall not miss the pleasure we would have experienced.

He cites a 19th century writer, Henry Salt[16], who in his *Animals' Rights* said:

> The fallacy lies in the confusion of thought that attempts to compare existence with non-existence. A person who is already in existence must feel that he would rather have lived than not, but he must first have the *terra firma* of existence to argue from; the moment he begins to argue as if from the abyss of the non-existent, he talks nonsense, by predicating good or evil, happiness or unhappiness, of that of which we can predicate nothing.

The cultural commentator Paul Carter draws on a complex argument by J Hillis Miller, the American literary critic.[17] Carter says:

> Hillis Miller has pointed out that one etymology for diegesis, the narration of events, gives as the word's original meaning the redrawing of a line already drawn. Plotting, in this context, is the desire to bring out the meaning of that line, to endow it with form, to bend it perhaps into the ring of eternal return.

We need to consider this idea carefully. For in giving the space that death occupies narrative form the individual may give life its fully-realized meaning.

We confront faith and belief, choice and autonomy (including the troubling distinction between precedent and contemporary autonomy – that is, can we act on a person's prior decisions made when competent, now that they are no longer so?) We make ethical judgements where we deal with the idea that we might be better off dead. When we consider euthanasia and autonomy, we should ask how strong is our commitment to autonomy, which Henry Thoreau, Robert Paul Wolff and others have located as 'the primary obligation of man' – an idea rejected by other spiritual critics.[18] Does respect for the value of autonomy support a judgement by an individual that longer life may not in every circumstance outweigh all other considerations, including sanctity? Does highly valuing autonomy require enabling the individual to judge their own tolerance of distress? We know that doctors cannot measure pain meaningfully, and that pain is a matter for individual endurance and assessment. Only the individual knows what is acceptable. Only the individual can say how much they can endure of vomiting, pain, intubation, the side-effects of cancerous growths which disable eating, sleeping, bowel control and poor breathing. These are among the reasons addressed by those seeking to die. Do we thus endorse the acts of the conscious individual who wishes to maintain control of themselves, and their dignity – even despite the fact that this will breach the sanctity of life ethic, it being over-ridden by self-determination? If we accept that the principle of autonomy requires us to allow rational agents to live as they wish, un-coerced – and if a rational individual autonomously chooses to die – then respect for autonomy would favour assistance in euthanasia within strictly controlled procedures. For, even admitting Henry Salt's gaunt and desolate logical helplessness, it is not *a priori* clear that we necessarily do harm if we support a personal judgement to die. Here, too, it is not an ethical decision to make no decision; it is an ethical responsibility to make decisions.

We have, too, to be sensitively aware of what people want before they ever reach the point that they may wish to die. One key is much better palliative care and greater investment in its benefits. Another is informed advance statements of preference and intent, with individual wishes expressed in writing. Both – that is, better palliative care and the option of expressing a wish in advance – could engage the patient in truly informed control over what happens to them, and especially in supporting them at home, which is so often the place of personal choice. This requires improved community services, making palliative care available wherever they may be. Such care, too, leads us in making up other deficits, particularly concerning communications and links between adjacent professions. It can lead the way in enabling individual autonomy and greater self-respect. It can, too, enhance understanding that the autonomy of the individual has a context, particularly that of the family and of the local community. It is clearly an ethical requirement that people are enabled to live in physical ease, in close personal relationships and are afforded the possibilities of emotional and spiritual growth whilst receiving treatment. This support is clearly influential in determining the quality of lives, the length of active life, and the ability to respond to specialist care. Better palliative care, too, impacts not only on coping-strategies with cancer but on the fears of the elderly of the burdens of extreme old age, dementia and helplessness.[19]

One requirement of great importance is that the degree of choice and of palliative support is evident, and that decisions concerning treatments are fully informed ones. This insists on an investment in symptom control, in effective consultation and communication. It asks, too, for measures to support the quality of life for a dying person and their family. This is very evidently not the same as voluntary euthanasia. Equally, this important commitment, which is much needed, does not of itself necessarily exclude such a choice, if that became legally available.

We know, of course, that there are those who offer palliative care and who are anxious that euthanasia should not be considered as a logical part or an extension of palliative care. These are clearly distinct ideas. Palliative care offers the recognition that the relief of suffering is often – and should be – the primary objective. We are not, indeed, all as fortunate as the Mother, whose end is described in Larry Watson's novel of childhood, *Montana 1948*: 'She made, as the expression goes, a good death. She came inside the house from working in her garden, and a heart attack, as sudden as a sneeze, felled her in the kitchen'. More typical for many more is the end of his other parent: 'My father's death, ten years earlier, was less merciful. Cancer hollowed him out over the years, until he could not stand up to a stiff wind'.[20]

This recognition of the importance of palliative care can co-exist, too, with the idea that the pursuit of a cure by aggressive medicine can be a distasteful and undignified illusion which itself imposes unnecessary pain. The responsibility is not only to consider individual choice as to whether to go on or not. It is also to bring relief of suffering to the vulnerable and to support them in living. It seems unarguable, too, that the availability of good palliative care and effective relief to improve the quality of the life remaining will itself influence attitudes to wanting to go on or not. Rationing intrudes here, as priorities press; we must get the priorities in the kindest balance.

When we face decisions which draw a life to a close how do we make an account of the value of the loss of life – how to assess and balance its duration, quality, impact on others, how to gauge the avoidance of pain, the loss of pleasures and relationships? Our terms of reference can constantly bifurcate unless we hold to an ethics in lived experience as a guide to baffling change. We are, much of the time, all migrants from our roots. In a world of delusive representations, contingency and difficulty in communications our answers require us to think *for ourselves* and to focus on the relationships of meaning between life and death.

We struggle for satisfactory answers where nothing fully satisfactory can be found. On these issues I take a broadly utilitarian position. We are confronting incompatible and incommensurable goods. For, as Isaiah Berlin says, 'Certain human values cannot be combined, because they are incompatible with one another'.[21] We have to make afflicted and often wretched choices, and we need a structure of ethical and moral principles by which to do so. We seek, of course, a close match between words, and feelings, in laying the stress on living. We seek, too, to help people find the strength to turn their own psychic life inside out. Thus, in moments of self-revelation in a succession of life events, they can find themselves as their guide.

Life is biographical as well as merely biological. For the unconscious patient who can never recover, is it wrong to allow such a patient – as in the Tony Bland and the Nancy Cruzan cases – to die?[22] Is it wrong, even if we judge that to die is in their best interests? Even though death inflicts a loss do we necessarily do wrong if we release a conscious and informed patient who asks to be released under carefully established provisions? Our need for a revising law and a rejuvenated ethics obliges us to consider whether in the case of the conscious patient, is it wrong to help a conscious person to die, if they wish such a course? Should the law allow doctors to kill terminally ill patients who plead to die? If we take the view that it should not do so, we do not escape from the realm of moral problems. For a moral problem remains: is it ethically wrong to inflict pain or to allow it to continue by refusing euthanasia? Should the law allow doctors not to treat patients suffering irreversible dementia or from cancer?

Nor do we necessarily do wrong if we release a patient in a coma whose cortex has been destroyed. For it has been medically-held that such a patient has no hope of recovery into normal life and no prospect of being able to see themselves again as existing over time. The Bland judgement gave this legal space and force. The vegetative or the coma patient is not in a voluntary situation. It is society (or the doctors, or the family, or the courts) which asks whether it is in the best interests of a patient in a permanent coma to be kept alive technologically. However, for the choices society might open to the conscious patient, we each need to make up our own minds. The problem of involuntary euthanasia is much more difficult and dangerous – critically, intuitively, morally.

We continue to face the choice between absolute and relative values. Does respect for the sanctity and inviolability of life embody our absolute duty to prolong life in all circumstances? These cases opened out a fundamental discussion of what it now means to be dead or not to be dead, what it is to be or not to be alive. What is it to be a person. Teresa Iglesias asks:

> If my body is 'instrumental' to what I am, if I am not really my body, what am I? If my body is 'my property' who is that non-bodily I that owns it?

I would put it similarly as follows: who is that who, who asks who is that who is looking at me in the mirror in the morning? Medical and social concepts of what it is to be a human being were thus challenged and examined. So, too, were the basic ideas which themselves constitute the nature of medicine, and these remain under pressure. The central commitment of the medical profession to the idea that our living identity is constituted precisely by our integrity and organization as one self-sustaining living and unified whole (whatever else a human being may be, in spiritual terms), was an essential pivot for discussions in court.

Most of us accept that life has an intrinsic sanctity. This is an essential social bond. Life is not merely narrowly instrumental, experiential or personal – although these are in themselves important values. It is not necessary to be religious to be spiritual (as Dickens shows in his Preface to *Barnaby Rudge*) or to be able to express individual moral opinions and to honour the sanctity of life. A commitment to the inviolability and sanctity of life is essential to the realization of the potential of individual lives. This is so, too, in considering those grave moral questions concerning those who are no longer (or who have never been) competent to reach their own decisions. Yet we disagree trenchantly, often violently, in defending sanctity. We disagree about what it is proper to do to alleviate suffering, and whether or not it is to be relieved at all costs. Commentators, indeed, disagree about what it is that constitutes 'suffering'.[23]

Our most emotional debates revolve around how we interpret sanctity in actual life situations. Our shared commitment to the sanctity of life is itself the source of our disagreements as to how to show respect to that commitment. For in making ethical decisions our individual interpretation of these intrinsic values fosters these divisions, lightens or darkens our lives. As CL Stevenson put this, our ethical judgements *express* our attitudes, rather than *describe* them. We disagree about ethics (which itself implies that it carries with it something bigger than the individual) *because* we try to express our attitude, to bring our listeners or readers to a similar attitude.[24]

RM Hare and his pupil Peter Singer both say that ethical judgements are prescriptions.[25] Our point of view resonates across the spectrum of our lives. For it is here that we seek to affirm life, curtail suffering and endorse autonomy which is the capacity to choose, to make and act on one's own decisions. We seek, too, to do something else, which is that we seek to interpret the best interests of others in special circumstances. This is one area where we get into great difficulties. In making our own decisions, and in making decisions in what we conceive to be the best interests of others, we employ three key concepts. These concern how we respect our own, or the patient's, autonomy, how we protect our own, or the patient's, best interests and how we protect the intrinsic sanctity or value of life.

We are in the territory of taboo, but one in which curtains are being lifted. We seek to make moral sense of confused debate, rife with misunderstandings. Here, too, we find people in similar circumstances making contradictory decisions. Frequently, these divergences are made by appeal to *shared* ethical and moral standards. Some seek to leave their lives, to leave behind extreme pain. Some choose to endure, even in what to others are unacceptable circumstances. The clue here is surely to understand that individuals are not only taking a view about the relative dreadfulness of what is likely to happen to them next. Instead, they are taking a view about what has happened to them in life. They wish to take account of who they have been and how they have realized their selves.

If we consider the difficulties from this quoin we can appreciate that death itself has a retrospective meaning. How death is managed itself is part of the character, and hence celebration or diminution, of life itself. This is to understand that an individual may not merely judge life as a succession of incremental details, but as a complete picture which includes death. Life is not merely, in the words of AJP Taylor 'one damn thing after another'. It is a *structure*, a whole whose value and completeness is both represented and encapsulated by the nature of its ending. This idea may be a best guide to how we need to think of autonomy on the death-bed. For we each need to choose how to cope at the end. We may expect more freedom. On this view, each experience and each moral decision is not a fragment. It is a prism for the whole. The Australian explorer Ludwig Leichhardt wrote of one of his outback travels: 'At the latter part of my journey, I had, as it were, retraced the whole course of my life'.[26] Such an idea relates fundamentally to how we each choose to live, to give meaning to our lives, to take responsibility for ourselves. We may be able to construct for ourselves an ethic and a morality in harnessing the scarcest resource in the world – the days (including especially the last days) of our lives.

In more than one sense, death is inescapable. We have, in my view, an individual responsibility of self-realization. We each have to respond ethically to the challenge to make our life worthwhile. There is, thus, a logical and ethical connectivity. How to live is inexplicable without a conviction of how to die. How to round out this mortal coil itself resonates with the nature of our intrinsic value in life itself. Equally, in the novelist Thomas Eidson's words, 'the world is not outside, it is in your head ... inside the one mind of the spirit. All things are within ... Life must be affirmed'.[27]

Purpose

This short work is thus about purpose. It is a personal exploration of delicate, enigmatical, difficult questions in ethics. It reflects, too, their application to fundamentals in health benefit. It began as a lecture. I have only tentatively and uneasily expanded it beyond those reassuring limits. It is, however, framed with some foundational convictions. These are essential, especially in this too often abstract and donnish area of discussion (where some questions are even too ambiguous to be useful). Most evidently, it offers a framework for endorsing individual self-realization in which we both seek to live a good life and also find it so. It argues for self-creation, self-responsibility and self-reflection in active command of our own lives, which include our deaths. In doing so, I try to suggest ways of considering some controverted issues – notably voluntary and involuntary euthanasia, dementia, the persistent vegetative state, and a cluster (and cloister) of questions concerned with killing or not killing.

I am, at the same time, aware that these arguments have a spiritual and a political context. It is these prompts which shapes them. For ethics must succeed in the academy, in the political forum and in the private heart. I suggest that these enigmatical issues are amenable to reasoning, and to accommodation in good conscience between opposing points of view. There is here, too, a most cardinal, central and constitutional point which we need to keep in view from every promontory. This is whether, as I have said, any political community ought to constitute itself to make intrinsic values a matter of collective decision. I agree with Dworkin: not.

My ambitions here are limited to a sketch. This work is not a comprehensive account of these critical moral and political questions. Others since Socrates (and, among our contemporaries, notably Ronald Dworkin, Peter Singer and, tangentially, Isaiah Berlin) have offered that. I follow Dworkin in the central argument that there needs to be choice and autonomy, together with understanding of why people disagree, notably in interpreting sanctity. I ride with him in accepting an important idea on horse-back: each part of our life is part of every part. How we live influences how we wish to die. How we die reflects on how we have lived, in self-realization and in dignity. I follow Singer in wishing to see a new ethics constructed which responds to changes in culture and medicine. He seems to me to be right, too, to seek to extend the reach and content of ethical conversations into environmental issues, although I do not explore these here.

Euthanasia is perhaps the most controversial and difficult ethical issue. This is in part because decisions about death can themselves have a greater dominion over life. Those who wish to be purposeful at the end, if at all possible, express a judgement about how they have lived, and how they wish to be thought of once they are gone. This notion asks for a conception both of life and of death which has integrity, one that is coherent with the ways in which individual lives have been lived. That is to say that people wish to die as they live, in character. We need to be wary, cautious and open here to the detailed concerns of those affected by change, particularly the elderly, terminally-ill patients and those with slight or serious dementia. Different people do, of course, take different views on how they wish to face and resolve death as an integral part of their personal drama. But the point, I think, is that it is the individual who can best determine their best interests as to the manner of their death. It is the individual who should seek to shape this in the manner of their life and their personal sense of their critical interests and concerns. This is to ask for the individual to be enabled to make choices about such care provision, or to clearly direct their relatives or carers as to their wishes. It is not to ask for coercion, for or against voluntary euthanasia. It is, however, in a sense, to take self-reliance beyond the grave by not regarding death as the disconnecting event alone, but as a connector of the whole of the life. This is, however, to deny that the personal is necessarily political. The role of politics should be to release the personal, in a kind and supportive regulatory framework.

This is to emphasize our responsibility for constructing our own moral lives. Those who share this view naturally wish the expressive manner of their deaths to be part of the statement which has characterized their lives. My touchstone here, and the essential pivot, is a key and brilliant passage by Ronald Dworkin, in his *Life's Dominion*. This makes the most essential point in all these debates:

> It is a platitude that we live our whole lives in the shadow of death; it is also true that we die in the shadow of our whole lives. Death's central horror is oblivion – the terrifying, absolute dying of the light. But oblivion is not all there is to death; if it were, people would not worry so much about whether their technical, biological lives continue after they have become unconscious and the void has begun, after the light is already dead forever. Death has dominion because it is not only the start of nothing but the end of everything, and how we think and talk about dying – the emphasis we put on dying with 'dignity' – shows how important it is that life ends *appropriately*, that death keeps faith with the way we want to have lived.

We needs must die, but not necessarily be dead in what Dickens calls 'a common sort of way'. Not, that is, if death is 'but a notch in the quiet calendar of a well-spent life', and if we can be 'in a green old age: at peace with [ourselves], and evidently disposed to be so with all the world'.[28]

Life and death decisions rest on two linked foundations: the belief in the intrinsic and sacred value of life, on the one hand, and the personal and individual value for the person as a life being lived, on the other. These foundations offer both a mystical and a secular discourse. But this does not necessarily require us to dilute the autonomy of the individual. Indeed, the contrary is true: the expression of self-realization in the individual may itself re-enforce our commitment to the sanctity of life, and to a good death which echoes both the self-realization and sanctity of these twinned foundations. To understand why people disagree on these ethical constructs – about abortion, euthanasia, autonomy – we need to be clear what it is that death means to people. We need greater understanding of what different ways of living their lives and dying their deaths mean to different people. It seems clear that for an increasing number the question of how to die is in part the question of how to live well.

The greatest of all minds, Francis Bacon (Viscount Verulam), opens his brief essay *Of Death* by telling us that 'Men fear death as children fear to go in the dark, and as that natural fear in children is increased with tales, so is the other'. The actor Paul Newman I recall says somewhere, with cryptic compression, that 'Nobody gets out of life alive'. It is little comfort, perhaps, that the great Tudor Lord Chancellor and poet reflected that the end has advantages: 'Death has this also, that it openeth the gate to good fame, and extinguisheth envy'.[29] Nor that elsewhere he adds the modernist understanding that 'no man knows his own death'. Indeed, increasingly, people wish to do so, in part as a test of knowing their own life and its shaping. However, aphorisms focus but do not banish dilemmas.

Intuitively, most of us believe that no-one could be better off dead, until we examine the quandaries and the painful circumstances that arise in so many lives. Intuitively, we think it must be bad to die, even if one is permanently unconscious. For even then how could being dead be an improvement for the individual concerned? None are indifferent to death, not even the suicide. Yet once a full life has been lived, Jonathan Swift argues in *Gulliver's Travels,* it is death itself which gives meaning to life. Here, the Dean suggested that without death existence would be merely gratuitous. So one of the objectives is to seek to invest both life and death with greater, fuller, connected meanings.

There are ethical philosophers who argue that heroically maintaining life in some cases itself causes the individual more damage than letting them go, especially when the individual has wished to avoid the 'benefits' of 'aggressive medicine'. Francis Bacon, on his unexpected Highgate death-bed, is reported to have said that 'I now enter on my usual condition'. Yet many of our ethical dilemmas focus on the inevitable fact of the oblivion of death by asking what it is to live a good life, including a 'good death'. This is to ask questions about the quality of the life already lived, the quality and integrity of the life remaining and of the wish of many individuals to exert control over the nature, locale, and time-frame of their own deaths with dignity and with understanding.

Citizens

Ronald Dworkin, with the poets, says that we should focus on life's dominion rather than on death's. For he holds up to our view 'the devastatingly important truth that what death means hinges on how and why our lives are sacred'.[30] This is where we make the most difficult choices as people and the most sensitive laws as citizens. We are concerned to draw defensible and workable lines, taking full account of many detailed and identifiable risks in articulating moral rights. It is, too, where we surely disagree very deeply precisely because, as Dworkin says, we are so alike. For each of us takes so very seriously the fundamental value which unites us as humans – that life is sacred at every stage. We differ over interpretations and actions – over the status of the fetus, the treatment of those suffering from dementia, the patient in a coma, the suffering person seeking euthanasia – because of the complexities of these values and the necessarily individual nature of self-realization. We differ, often excitedly, too, in the priority we give to absolute values, in how individuals and cultures interpret what 'sacred' means, and from which sources it derives.

It seems correct to say that we disagree so fundamentally about solutions because we agree so passionately about the sanctity of the questions. For whichever choices are made are a celebration of the sanctity of life. This is not an area of disputation, however, in which mutual and tolerant understanding is usual. It is one where many suspect all motives except their own. However, it is important to acknowledge that the common value in the different choices people make is respect for human and individual dignity and self-respect (with which dignity is integral). For we seek to act on life and death questions in order to express the intrinsic value of life and of life's dominion. Self-respect rounds out our lives. It is the spirit of our lives and of our decisions concerning death.

We need to understand these quandaries in interpretation if we are to balance the rival risks and hazards of public policies on life and death questions, to make decisions as individuals and as citizens. Most of us seek to structure our lives around good experiences and reasoned and judicious choices which turn on the polar axis of our dignity and self-respect. We can be united by our commitment to the sanctity of life as a fundamental value and thus locate precisely the reasons why we disagree. For, to exemplify, one interpretation and one expression of respect will encourage a rational individual to seek a quick and peacefully dignified death. Yet another will fight to the last breath. Many who are in very great and unrelievable pain wish to die whilst they are still competent to arrange it, control it and know it is happening. Many dread the vegetative state and fear remaining technologically alive but dead within themselves.

Doctors manage these situations differently now. Some terminally-ill patients are allowed to slip away. Others have been helped to do so. In the UK, none may legally ask to be helped to die. There are many delicate, difficult, legal, medical and moral issues here. There are, too, irrational lines drawn which seem to generate suffering as well as solace. The distinction, for example, between a directly intended-effect and an unintended (but expected?) side-effect looks contrived and doubtful. Responsibility surely adheres to both categories of action. Similarly unsatisfactory is the distinction between 'ordinary' and 'extraordinary' treatments and their justifications. Here, allowing a patient to die does not seem morally different from actively assisting a patient to die. Indeed, it may be *less* humane in itself passively to hold back and to let disease take its course.

Can we sustain the distinction summarized in the 'acts and omission' doctrine widely used by doctors to justify withholding life-saving treatments in circumstances where they would condemn killing a patient but where t death from natural causes (perhaps in extremes of pain) would acceptable? Or is this a thin line with no moral substance? That is ethical distinction between active and passive euthanasia? And, *e* is not, are the risks of the latter too great because of the social consequences? For example, in the impact on attitudes towards medicine and in attitudes towards themselves amongst the elderly and vulnerable. There are many cases of terminal cancer where life-prolonging antibiotics are withheld from a patient who develops pneumonia. New-born infants with severe defects may or may not receive active treatment. Is this more acceptable morally than actively administering a lethal overdose which has identical, predictable, painless results? British law says yes. Passive action is permissible; active action is direct killing and illegal. Utilitarians find this an unsatisfactory position of no moral value. Others say that this distinction may not be defensible as a morally valid principle, but that there are features associated with it that are of moral significance. Thus, it is better to have a general moral prohibition against killing but only a weak injunction against people being allowed to die. This may support practices that provide a necessary basis for trust between patients and professionals offering care, which should be equivalent to benefit. We are offered the fear of the slippery slope; we are offered a social institution; we are not offered a defensible moral principle.[31]

One may think it irrational to be allowed to insist on dying slowly by refusing help but not be enabled to ask for help to die less slowly when in the grossest pain. People may wish to avoid a lingering, painful, technological death – being biologically alive but gripped in a treatment regime of indignity, medical heroism and a lack of respect for how the individual has lived. Another will wish to honour that sanctity by saving every second despite its quality. Ethics presently allow letting die but not aiding death. Doctors seem to make illogical decisions in distinguishing between active and passive euthanasia. It may be that medical intuition cannot be captured in formal ethical principles, as a central part of moral reasoning. In health care ethics, however, we must provide a more secure basis for moral decisions than the intuition of doctors and nurses. We need an ethical basis for what intuitively we may regard as common-sense. The distinction between acts and omissions is difficult to defend.[32]

I am persuaded that the manner of dying is integral to the self-respect of life. Many believe that controlling how they die is the most respectful expression of their belief in the sanctity and inviolability of life itself. These individuals evidently take the view that to remain alive in some circumstances is more harmful than to be helped to die, although those of us not facing this awful choice (or only prospectively) may feel that nothing can be worse than non-existence.

There are, too, social issues on which we need to place weight, including the integrity of the doctor as a moral agent and other safeguards for the vulnerable (who may fear being killed, who may become anxious that the protective role of health professionals may change and who may be concerned at what may happen to them once incompetent). However, it seems to me that Dworkin is correct to write:

> the question posed by euthanasia is not whether the sanctity of life should yield to some other value, like humanity or compassion, but how life's sanctity should be understood and respected.

I find this a persuasive account and a guide to conduct. For decisions are individually needed both about one's personal rights and best interests and about how society can most successfully re-emphasize the importance of the intrinsic value of human life.

I mentioned foundational convictions. There are here some liberal assumptions about what we mean by being a person and what a society should represent. Most notably, the objective is to support and enable individual self-realization, self-creation, self-responsibility and self-reflection in active command of our own lives. For we shape and re-shape our lives as we discover ourselves, as we express our individual, and sometimes 'irrational', personality. Here is the notion of the integrity of the individual made evident in the integrity of informed choice, even if we would not ourselves have made the particular medical or non-medical choices others make. This offers the framework that competent adults have a right to autonomy by which they can make those important life-defining decisions for themselves. It is this autonomy which is so often at stake in medical contexts, where rights are most discussed, amended, limited and interpreted in our 'best interests' by others.

Professor Dworkin is surely right to say:

> Decisions about life and death are the most important, the most crucial for forming and expressing personality, that anyone makes; we think it crucial to get these decisions right, but also crucial to make them in character, and for ourselves.[33]

This is where individual action and public policy must be located. It is where the critical foundations lie for self-realization in self-consciousness, self-respect and the sources of the sanctity of life. It is where we say that each of us has critical interests which express the value of each life for its own sake. It is where we can eventually come to our dreadful day when we each may make a statement about finality which gives meaning to everything. This is to suggest that each of us can best hope to have individual moral standing in the moral community. For how we die in all possible dignity itself re-affirms the importance of our individual life – *up to and including death and its course.* This pervasive and central recognition is important, for it expresses both the intrinsic sanctity of human life and also its individual value. It is this dual sacredness for which I urge respect. It is this duality which needs recognition as we consider difficult ethical choices, in the Kantian sense that we are ends in ourselves and not means.

Staring

It is both subjectively and objectively important how a life is lived and how it ends. This is so for the individual and for society. La Rochefoucauld, as Dworkin reminds us, said that death, like the sun, should not be stared at.[34] Yet without doing so we may not be able to see life and its potentials, nor understand that the most vital concern is self-realization.

These complex, and often venomously controverted, questions require us all to reflect, to reason and to make sense for ourselves. Then to act as persons and as citizens. The position will become much more complex, and quickly too. Technology, which is itself political, increases urgency. We are only at the beginning of the challenges that science and technology will bring, as nanotechnology and computing proffer the re-design of 'life' in its fundamentals. Indeed, further on (but perhaps not too far further) our descendants may be a symbiotic neural network of organic and artificial components. They may thus transmute the very meaning of the words 'death' and 'life', 'person' and 'choice'. Then they will need a new ethics of their own. As Peter Davies has said:

> With the development of nanotechnology, the distinction be-
> tween living and nonliving, natural and artificial, brain and
> computer, will become increasingly blurred.[35]

This is anguishing personal, political, metaphysical and religious territory. Here both logic and illogic find their niches. This is a terrain where theoretical analysis of intricate personal problems is not necessarily satisfying or always helpful, either, in making real individual decisions. However, it must be appropriate to seek to construct a basis of understanding and of action. Here, we can ask how much choice builds a good society, and if there may be special areas where choice can disintegrate lives. This is the hearth and home of both fine and clumsy, helpful and un-necessary distinctions; of the puzzling and the paradoxical; of the intolerant and the magnanimous. This fireside is crowded with interests, rights and rhetoric. It is where we find morally problematic questions, including whether these should be in question at all. Yet it is common ground that is necessary to construct a moral and ethical code to live by if life is to have meaning and if society is to be a society. Coherence requires that such a code receives general consent and that within the code there is not only the potential for civil disagreement and for development and response, but also for individual conscience.

The most vigorous clashes in these debates (often in spiritual language) come from differing interpretations and from variant views of whether or not society will seek to coerce individuals or alternatively leave them to express their own responsibility. This is where we are in difficulties if we seek to ordain, coerce, enjoin and appoint a collective and political judgement on individuals who may wish to make such decisions in the light of their own spiritual and personal convictions. Put bluntly: is it for the state to define us, or is this the responsibility of ourselves? Are these to be relationships of control or of self-reflection? Further, if the emphasis is instead to be on self-responsibility (which cannot be commanded, or delivered politically), what are the grounds for exceptions and why? The cross-examination of such a question as 'Who owns our bodies?' captures those subjects which mark 'the edges of life'. We need to ask what these debates are *really* about and how might first principals be established which would form the ethical and moral code by which each of us may be able to live?

Miss Miggs, in *Barnaby Rudge*, with her sighing, sideways looks, told us:

> 'we never know the full value of some wines and fig-trees till we lose 'em. So much the worse, sir, for them as has the slighting of 'em on their consciences when they're gone to be in full blow elsewhere'. And Miss Miggs cast up her eyes to signify where that might be.[36]

Whether we will be in 'full blow' or not, which is Hope and which is Anchor, which is presage and which foreboding, Dickens leaves us to consider. For this is the larger frame, which complicates these discussions – the key reference point – whether the Universe and life has any meaning, and if it has how we might come to know it.

People bring their idiosyncratic answers to these cosmic questions. In such a difficult dominion lie the most difficult and complex personal, ethical, moral, social, political and religious quandaries. It is here that we constantly bump into such baffling and foxy concepts as 'sanctity', 'intrinsic value', 'dignity' (and the right to avoid indignity), 'beneficence', 'competence', 'duty' and 'autonomy'. Hamlet the Prince understood this most troublingly of us all. As the King says with such under-statement, 'there's matter in theese sighes'.[37]

Notes

1   I am especially beholden to the landmark work by Ronald Dworkin – Dworkin R (1993) *Life's dominion: an argument about abortion and euthanasia*. Alfred A Knopf, New York. I do not, however, address in

detail the complete range of conditions and issues he addresses. For example, abortion or dementia. I refer the reader to his discussion, which I find a wholly persuasive account of the nature of those debates, of why they matter, of why people disagree and of the appropriate responses. I have also found especially valuable Singer P (1995) *Rethinking life and death: the collapse of our traditional ethics*. OUP, Oxford (first published in 1994 by the Text Publishing Company, Melbourne), and his bibliography. See also discussions in Thomson JJ (1971) In defence of abortion. *Philosophy & Public Affairs* **1**(1) and Tooley M (1972) Abortion and infanticide. *Philosophy & Public Affairs* **2**(1), both reprinted in Singer P (ed.) (1986) *Applied ethics*. OUP, Oxford.

2   John Locke's definition of 'person' is in Locke J (1690) *Essay concerning human understanding*. Book 1, Chapter 9, Paragraph 29.

3   See Dworkin, *ibid*. Also Dworkin R (1977) *Taking rights seriously*. Duckworth, London, and Singer P (1995), op.cit. See also Singer P (ed.) (1986), op.cit., especially James Rachels, *Active and passive euthanasia*, first published in 1975 in *NEJM* **292**: 78–80; Singer P (1993) (2nd ed.) *Practical ethics*. CUP, Cambridge; Singer P (ed.) (1994) *Ethics*. OUP, Oxford.

4   See Sterne L (1759–67) *The life and opinions of Tristram Shandy, Gentleman*. Volume viii, Chapter 2; Volume i, Chapter 1 from line one onwards.

5   See Strong C (1991) Fetal tissue transplantation: can it be morally insulated from abortion? *J. Med. Ethics* **17**: 70–6, and Brecher B (1991) Buying human kidneys: autonomy, commodity and power. *J. Med. Ethics* **11**: 99.

6   See Pickering W (1991) A nation of people called patients. *J. Med. Ethics* **17**: 91–2, and Pickering W (1996) Is the word 'patient' in the way of better care? In: *Patients' Voices*. The Patients Association, London.

7   The Gothick imagery is prevailing. For example, Mary Shelley in Hindle M (ed.) (1992) *Frankenstein, or the modern Prometheus*. Classics edition. Penguin, London.

8   William Shakespeare, *Richard II*, Act 5, scene 5.

9   See Singer P (1995), op.cit., especially Chapter 8, *Beyond the discontinuous mind*, and Singer P (1993), op.cit., especially Chapter 5, *Taking life: animals*.

10   Holy Bible, King James Version, *Genesis*, 1: 24–8.

11   See Singer P (1993), op.cit., especially Chapter 3, *Equality for animals?*

12   Carter P (1992) *Living in a new country: history, travelling and language*. Faber & Faber, London, pp. 19 and 23.

13 Vincent JR (1976) (2nd ed.) *The formation of the British Liberal Party, 1857–1868.* The Harvester Press, Brighton.

14 WB Yeats, cited by A Alvarez (1986), in the introduction to *Laurence Sterne, a sentimental journey through France and Italy.* Classics edition. Penguin, London. I owe the Empson reference, from his poem *Dissatisfaction with metaphysics,* to the introduction by Christopher Ricks to Sterne L (1986) *Tristram Shandy.* Classics edition. Penguin, London.

15 It is, of course, a matter of belief. There are those who face death as if this is an expedition of discovery and renewal, like a child in a boat. The quotations from William Shakespeare are in *The Tempest,* Act 4, scene 1; *Hamlet,* Act 3, scene 1. Peter Singer's comment on death is in *Practical ethics* (1993), op.cit., p. 102, as is his surprising but persuasive discussion of species membership, especially Chapters 3, 4, and 5.

16 See Henry Salt, *Animals' rights,* cited in Singer P (1993) *Practical ethics, ibid.,* p. 122.

17 J Hillis Miller is cited by Carter P (1992), op.cit., from Brooks P (1984) *Reading from the plot.* OUP, Oxford, p. 21.

18 The quotation from Robert Paul Wolff is in Wolff RP (1970) *In defence of anarchism,* cited by Singer P (1993), op.cit., p. 292 where he also discusses Henry Thoreau's ideas.

19 See Saunders C (1992) Voluntary euthanasia. *Palliative Medicine* 6: 1–5. But see also Haas F (1994) In the patient's best interests? Dehydration in dying patients. *Professional Nurse* 10(2): 82–7, which queries care that often causes patients distress in the final stages of their illness. Chalmers GL (1985) Ethical conflicts in the long term care of aged patients: a response. *Ethics & Medicine* 1(4): 58–60, discusses the problem of variation according to the fluctuations in feeling and opinion of the individual patient in decision-making, and the need for a reference to an ethic which is beyond either pragmatism or subjectivism.

20 See Watson L (1995) *Montana 1948: a novel.* Macmillan, London.

21 See Isaiah Berlin, in Jahanbegloo R (1992) *Conversations with Isaiah Berlin: recollections of an historian of ideas.* Peter Halbon, London.

22 See *Airedale NHS Trust v. Bland (CA),* 19 February 1993, 2 WLR 316–400 and *Cruzan v. Director, Missouri Department of Health* (1990) 110, Supreme Court, 2841. See especially the important paper by Iglesias T (1995) Ethics, brain-death and the medical concept of the human being. *Medico-legal Journal of Ireland* 1(2): 51–7. Also, Keown J (1993) Courting euthanasia? Tony Bland and the Law Lords. *Ethics & Medicine* 8: 3; Cranford RE (1988) The persistent vegetative

state: the medical reality (getting the facts straight). *Hastings Center Report* **18(1)**: 27–8; Lezak MD (1986) Psychological implications of traumatic brain damage for the patient's family. *Rehabilitation Psychology* **31**: 4.

The majority of legal opinions that comprised the judgement in the Tony Bland case emphasized the patient's best interests which prevailed against continuing treatment, rather than the patient's self-determination. See references which I cite in my further discussion of the Tony Bland case in my lecture. The discussions in Dworkin (1993), op.cit. and Singer (1965), op.cit. are especially helpful. Dworkin's discussion of constitutional issues are of particular importance in the American context, where he is Professor of Law at New York University, in addition to his Oxford appointment.

For another and different 'best-interests' case, where the Court of Appeal in London upheld the refusal of parents to consent to a life-saving liver transplant for their 18-month old son, see Bale J (1996) Mother wins right to stop surgery. In: *The Times*, 25 October 1996; Struttaford T (1996) Operation has good chance of success. In: *The Times*, 25 October 1996; Barwick S (1996) Parents must decide fate of liver boy, judges rule. In: *The Daily Telegraph*, 25 October 1996.

23   On these points see Cameron NM Rt Rev Dr (1985) New medicine for old. *Ethics & Medicine* **1**: 4.

24   See CL Stevenson, cited in Singer (1993), op.cit., p. 7.

25   See Hare RM (1952) *The language of morals*. OUP, Oxford; Hare RM (1963) *Freedom and reason*. Clarendon Press, Oxford; Hare RM (1991) Universal presciptivism. In: *A companion to ethics* (ed. P Singer). Blackwell, Oxford; Christman J (ed.) (1989) *The inner citadel: essays on individual autonomy*. OUP, New York; Rachels J (1986) *The end of life*. OUP, Oxford; Vardy P and Grosch P (1994) *The puzzle of ethics*. HarperCollins, London, offer a general survey.

26   Ludwig Leichardt, quoted in Carter (1992), op.cit., p. 16.

27   See Eidson T (1995) *The last ride*. Michael Joseph, London, p. 85.

28   See Dworkin R (1993), op.cit., p. 199. Also, Dickens C (1841) *Barnaby Rudge: a tale of the riots of 'eighty*. Chapman and Hall, London; Spence G (ed.) (1986) *Barnaby Rudge*. Classics edition. Penguin, London, pp. 53, 63.

29   See introduction by John Pitcher (1985) to *Francis Bacon: the essays*. Penguin, London.

30   Dworkin R (1993), op.cit., p. 238.

31   Johnson K (1993) A moral dilemma: killing and letting die. *British J. Nursing* 2 Dec 93, offers a helpful and balanced discussion. See also

the important paper by Rachels J (1975), op.cit. and Rachels J (1986), op.cit.; also Glover J (1977) *Causing death and saving lives*. Penguin, Harmondsworth; Harris J (1981) Ethical problems in the treatment of severely handicapped children. *J. Med. Ethics* 7: 117–21; Kuhse H and Singer P (1985) *Should the baby live?* OUP, Oxford. But see Gillon R (1988) Euthanasia, withholding life-prolonging treatment and the moral differences between killing and letting die. *J. Med. Ethics* **14**: 115–17. On the 'slippery slope', see Dworkin's dismissal of its confusions in Dworkin R (1993), op.cit., pp. 216–17, and Burgess J (1993) The great slippery slope argument. *J. Med. Ethics* **3**: 169–74.

32   See Johnson K (1993), *ibid.*, p. 636.

33   See Dworkin R (1993), op.cit., p. 239. On the anxieties of the vulnerable see, for example, the views in Cameron NM Rt Rev Dr (1985), op.cit.; Bexell G, Norberg A and Norberg B (1985) Ethical conflicts in long term care of aged patients. *Ethics & Medicine* **1**: 3; Chalmers GL (1985) Ethical conflicts in the long term care of aged patients: a response. *Ethics & Medicine* **1**: 4; Saunders C (1992), op.cit.; Johnson K (1993), op.cit. For a defence of moral absolutism derived from the Judaeo-Christian tradition and against the acceptance of moral relativism as state doctrine see, for example, Johnson P (1985) Withdraw this licence to kill. *Ethics & Medicine* **1**: 4.

34   See Dworkin (1993), op.cit., p. 237.

35   See Davies P (1994) *The last three minutes: conjectures about the ultimate fate of the universe*. Weidenfeld & Nicolson, London. See also, Kitcher P (1996) *The lives to come: the genetic revolution and human possibilities*. The Penguin Press, London. Singer's commentary *Taking life: animals* in Singer P (1993), op.cit., is a disturbing account of our placing of our species above the lives of members of other species.

36   Dickens C (1841), op.cit., pp. 267–8.

37   Shakespeare, *Hamlet*, Act 4, scene 2.

Who Owns Our Bodies?

'The truth's superb surprise'

Nearly 40 years ago the psychiatrist Erik Erikson[1] memorably described each patient as 'a universe of one'. In this spirit, I have chosen as my topic: Who owns our bodies? The answer is not obvious. Who owns our bodies? Whose life is it, anyway? How is this ownership to be expressed? This is the fundamental question of how to live, put in special terms. The answers may seem unsurprising, indeed intuitively obvious. But is this so?

I am trained as a historian, not as a professional philosopher. In this regularly ploughed philosophic meadow I cannot expect to be original, but I can try to be thoughtful. Nathaniel Hawthorne writes, in *The Blithedale Romance,* of 'those Lyceum-halls of which almost every village now has its own, dedicated to that sober and pallid, or rather drab-coloured, mode of winter-evening entertainment, the Lecture'.[2] We are of course in April, TS Eliot's 'cruellest month', yet I do feel a little like Hawthorne. For it was Henry James Sr who saw him at an idealist meeting in Boston and described him as looking 'like a rogue who finds himself in the company of detectives'.

My argument is that we do own our bodies, and that *choice* is the expression of ownership. Indeed, that choice is a value with special transforming powers which can only be evolved within oneself. My argument is that we should be the authors of our own self-transformations in life, since this builds genuine liberty. That we should not merely live passively with a stranger. That we should, instead, seek both self-knowledge and command. I argue, too, that the centrality of the *activity of choice* is itself uniquely transforming in self-development. Here, I follow Isaiah Berlin[3] and Friedrich Hayek[4] in being comfortable with the notion that choice is the basic element in our personal constitution, essential both for the individual resolution of moral dilemmas and for modern health care. However, it appears that we cannot achieve regeneration without pain, nor always find transformation without tragedy. And even the pilgrim fathers arrived in a snow storm.

We should seek, as JS Mill[5] urges, to express personal moral choices in terms of our own convictions. The role of the law should be to support this view but also, inevitably, to shape and contain it. Here modern medicine poses especially anguishing moral dilemmas. It may be, however, that here our hope for rational choice amongst moral dilemmas posed by medicine is too great a hope. That, as Berlin[3] suggests, the choices we face about life and death are increasingly posed as choices among irreconcilable and tragically difficult ends. For example – as current court cases show – choices about love: doing everything possible to sustain life, and reducing intolerable pain, but intruding on another's autonomy and sanctioning the end of someone else's life. For this collides with the value of individual choice and with Herzen's advice that, 'The ultimate goal of life is life itself'.[6]

There may be no appeal to absolutes, or to a principle of rights and liberty set out in contracts. It may be that Berlin[3] is right, and that we must hope for a system of consensus around conscience; in shared principles of decency as the basis to enable individuals to make agonized choices for themselves between incompatible goods. We know, of course, that cultures and choices are historically and culturally specific. Even our own times change.

The problem of whether or not there are 'natural rights' (and of how, if at all, they might be enforced) is a commonplace of philosophy. So, too, is the monist reliance for the one true answer on prescriptive authority, on revelation, on science, or on 'the Party'. We are instead asked to think culturally, to try to get to knowledge, and to truth (which is, of course, often different) by emphasizing choice.

Let us venture into these iceberged waters. We are considering moral dilemmas which we see in health care, and, more widely, the issue of citizen choice and empowerment. We should, in particular, perhaps concern ourselves with a cluster of cultural issues visible in daily work in the NHS. These concern possession and dispossession. These are at the heart of our cultural problem, in conceptualizing modern health care, not merely in obtaining it, or (as the official language goes) in 'delivering' it. The ways in which the NHS formulates questions, and its approved behaviours in practice, have a wide and often culturally damaging impact. We need, too, to recognize the knowledge, as Erving Goffman[7] noted and Malcolm Bradbury[2] has discussed, that social existence is itself a theatre in which individuals play multiple roles, assuming, presenting and disguising the self: 'Hence the self is hidden, ambiguous or simply the sum of the roles; social existence is a disguise, a masquerade, a ritual, a set of assigned activities'.

We have here the intersection of medicine, philosophy, law and of how each of us seeks to define ourselves. This is the landscape of goals, emotions, hopes, fears and expectations. It is, necessarily, one of anguished choices, imaginative visions, and all other forms of human experience. This is the territory of tragic challenges, between apparently irresolvable options, none of which are acceptable to the individual. In this locale confusion, bewilderment and division have arisen since, as Peter Singer[8] noted, 'After ruling our thoughts and our decisions about life and death for nearly two thousand years, the traditional western ethic has collapsed'.

Singer seeks, as do many, a compassionate, responsive, believable and more flexible ethical attitude which is defensible and which will replace the inherited moral architecture which seems no longer able to support anguished decisions. But these ethical decisions may necessarily remain anguished, seem arbitrary, and still lead us to outcomes that nobody wants. For, in his conversations with Ramin Jahanbegloo,[6] Berlin says:

> Some moral, social and political values conflict. I cannot conceive of any world in which certain values may be reconciled. I believe, in other words, that some of the ultimate values by which men live cannot be reconciled or combined, not just for practical reasons, but in principle, conceptually ... Justice and mercy, knowledge and happiness can collide. If that is true, then the idea of a perfect solution of human problems – of how to live – cannot be coherently conceived. It is not that such a perfect harmony cannot be created, because of practical difficulties, the very idea of it is conceptually incoherent. Utopian solutions are in principle incoherent and unimaginable. Such solutions want to combine the uncombinable. Certain human values cannot be combined, because they are incompatible with one another.

This is thus the human and clinical location where the most difficult, tormenting and sleepless moral questions reside. Those which look to be undecidable by rational reflection alone, or merely by 'authority', or technique, or logic. Berlin[3] comments, too, that, 'Philosophy comes from the collision of ideas which create problems. The ideas come from life. Life changes, so do the ideas, so do the collisions. The collisions breed puzzles ... the social changes ... breed new problems, the very idea that you can even in principle find solutions, is absurd.'

This is the area, too, as Langdon Winner[9] discusses, where the apparently inexhaustible power of scientific technology makes all things possible, and where it remains to be seen where the line is to be drawn, and how. Where the individual and society may wish to say that here are possibilities that it would be wise to avoid, that there are moral limits to technological change, that our best sense of who we are should guide us in decisions.

What, then, to do? Clearly, there have to be choices. Choices which can be very painful. I believe that Berlin[3] is right to advise that our only genuine prospect is the role of personal choice. And that the role of government and of the law is to protect choices from being too agonizing (as well as to protect choice as an activity in itself).

This means that we need a system which permits the pursuit of sometimes conflicting but pluralist values, so that, as far as possible, people do not find themselves in any situation which makes them do something contrary to their own deepest moral convictions. Even then, transparency and accountability is necessary, whilst coercion is avoided.

This is the territory of thought, feeling, behaviour and action, where ideas, beliefs, outlooks and the conflict of feelings and actions have to be dealt with by individuals themselves. These are about whether we are to define ourselves by reference to external factors, or from within, and in what balance between. Ethicists remind us that these questions are about the adequacy of the autonomous agent. Berlin[3] reminds us to ask what we mean by autonomy, by respect for the autonomy of others. This enquiry calls into question the authority of the law (and its ethnocentric social context). It implies, too, appraising the allocation of scarce resources and it prompts discussions of the claims of distributive justice. Above all, here is the question of the intrinsic value of human life and of value judgements about this. And of Berlin's reminder that history is all too full of the agonies of men who have tried to evade the tragic responsibility of choice by placing their faith in final and absolute truths.

A critical pivot in such discussions has been between so-called 'positive' liberty – seen as rational self-determination and autonomy, the freedom of self-mastery in life – and 'negative' liberty – seen as the absence of constraints imposed by others. 'Negative' here sounds more positive. For 'negative' liberty recognizes that the necessarily rivalrous diversity of human purposes and goods in ethical debates cannot be sorted out on the basis of a theory which offers principles to determine agonizing conflicts. Instead, choices must be made by individuals, in their own terms. Autonomy is not necessarily a prerequisite for this.

Lord Noel Annan[10] has commented here:

> Positive freedom is the benign name given to the theory which maintains that not merely wise philosophers but the state, indeed governments themselves, can identify what people would *really* want were they enlightened, if they possessed fully developed personalities and understood fully what was needed to promote a good, just and satisfying society. For if it is true that this can be identified then surely the state is justified in ignoring what ordinary people say they desire or detest ... People are often convinced by this vision of freedom because they want to believe in a commonsense view of goodness. Surely goodness must be

indivisible, surely truth is beauty and beauty truth, surely the different aspects of truth and goodness can always be reconciled. But Berlin declares that sometimes they cannot. Ideology answers the question 'How should I behave?' and 'How should I live?' People want to believe that there is one irrefutable answer to these questions. But there is not.

My own view is that freedom must be conceived in terms of the absence of constraints by others, with some legally agreed exceptions. Negative freedom, or choices among alternatives unobstructed by others, for preference. Philosophers, being complex in order to be clear, disagree about whether or not negative freedom must underpin the positive freedom of autonomy. This is a debate about whether autonomy designates rational choice among genuine options, or whether negative freedom only requires the basic freedom of choice as intrinsic and sufficient. Berlin, says Gray,[11] offers the idea that basic freedom of choice-making does not support the idea of autonomy, but of self-creation. That is, where the self is created without necessarily becoming an autonomous agent. Self-creation need not conform to an ideal of rational autonomy. For there are good lives (the nun, the soldier) which are not necessarily autonomous. Certainly, choice can be capricious and not rational and still embody basic freedom. So, seeking freedom and some concept of autonomy is not always easy to ground in philosophy or in practice, even if one does not seek to insist on an approved context for choice before allowing it.

Berlin[3] is the master in clarifying what is really at stake. He says:

> There are two separate questions. One is 'How many doors are open to me?'; the other is: 'Who is in charge here? Who is in control?' These questions are interwoven, but they are not the same, and they require different answers. How many doors are open to me? The question about the extent of negative liberty is to do with what obstacles lie before me. What am I prevented from doing by other people – deliberately or indirectly, unintentionally, or institutionally? The other question is: 'Who governs me? Do others govern me or do I govern myself? If others, by what right, what authority? If I have a right to self-rule, autonomy, can I lose this right? Can I give it away? Waive it? Recover it? In what way? Who makes the laws? Or implements them? Am I consulted? Does the majority govern? Why? Does God? The priests? The Party? The pressure of public opinion? Of tradition? By what authority?' Both questions, and their sub-questions, are central and legitimate. Both have to be answered ... Both are genuine questions. Both are inescapable. And the answers to them determine the nature of a given society.

John Gray[11] has recently summarized Berlin's 'single idea of enormous sub-
versive force', value-pluralism, together with Berlin's concept of 'agnostic
liberalism', which accepts a liberalism of conflict and unavoidable loss
amongst rivalrous goods and evils. This locates the grounds of many of the
difficulties of making choices about ethical dilemmas which medicine now
poses. That ultimate human values are objective but irreducibly diverse,
that they are conflicting and often uncombinable, and that sometimes when
they come into conflict with one another they are incommensurable; that is,
they are not comparable by any rational measure. Thus, the implication for
political philosophy – and of the moral dilemmas implied in the question
'Who owns our bodies?' – is that the idea of a perfect society in which all
genuine ideals and goods are achieved is both utopian and incoherent. This
stoic view looks like the reality we see in the newspapers, discussing 'right
to life' cases. It looks like the reality of unavoidable conflict and irreparable
loss, the tragedies we observe. We can see that this is the case when substituted
judgements have to be made about whether or not to keep someone alive.
Or when direct judgements have to be made: whether to end one's own life.

This is clearly our difficulty and our anguish in making ethical decisions in
the hope of reconciling incompatible ends, liberties and equalities. Ultimately, we may all wish to be empowered in terms of our own values and
beliefs in an increasingly pluralistic and relativist society. We require the
mechanisms, and the devices, to make this real. But we will still find ourselves
making decisions between necessarily conflicting ideals: to stay alive, but
without pain; to relieve suffering, but not take a life; to give our love, but
be unable to cope with the idea that we should end the life of a loved one. Who
owns our bodies opens up many issues of empowerment.

My chief theme focuses especially and primarily on the prismatic question
of whether society – and health systems – is inevitably to be experienced as
a network of controls, of hierarchical decision-making. Or whether 'ordinary'
people can be 'given' power, most notably within and over themselves. As
I have suggested, my context is that choice is a value with special transforming powers which can only be evolved *within* oneself. My argument is
that we should be the authors of our own self-transformations in life, since
this builds genuine liberty. That we should not merely live passively with
a stranger, but instead seek both self-knowledge and command, since the
centrality of the *activity of choice* is itself uniquely transforming in self-
development. It is the fulcrum of both life and death.

My view is that choice is the most basic of all freedoms. This is to rely on
Berlin's[3] account of 'negative' freedom conceived as the absence of constraints imposed by others, by contrast with a 'positive' account of freedom
where people are 'made' free, often by 'the State' or 'the Party'. My view of
the necessary development of, for example the NHS, is that a better society
and better health care can only come from individuals holding explicit

freedom rooted in self-responsibility. This is necessarily based in self-reflection, which uniquely builds self-esteem. This, too, in a real health system, which is primarily tax-based, universalist and which encompasses the vital moral imperative of better health care for the poor.

Who owns our bodies? This is clearly one of those misleadingly simple but imperious questions at which wise men and women take to their heels. But they should not flee. Nor, indeed, may we. St Augustine, amongst other authorities, says not. He puts it like this: 'Men go abroad to wonder at the height of mountains, at the huge waves of the sea, at the long courses of rivers, at the vast compass of the ocean, at the circular motion of the stars; and they pass by themselves without wondering.'

We should not pass by these dilemmas. For they will very likely enter each of our lives. We should wonder about the complexities of possible answers, and seek a moral guide to duty and conduct, but be aware of Berlin's[3] warnings that it is not possible to have everything. We need to think through these questions for a variety of relationships. For ourselves; for those we may have to care for; for those who may have to care for us; for those whom we will never know.

An area of special difficulty is also one of special possibility. For the fact that medicine and technology have blurred the distinction between being alive and being dead prompts us to think about these moral and social questions. This poses fundamental dilemmas. These are both cultural and political as well as medical and technical questions. And, most essentially, they are existential. For, as Gustave Flaubert wrote of doctors: 'They cannot find our souls with their scalpels'.[12] Medicine can now sustain the pulse of life without the individual gaining, or re-gaining, the potential to live a full life. But we are seeing something else, which is new. We are seeing what we mean by life and not-life being queried. We are seeing what we mean by death and not-death being doubted. We are at risk of re-defining this final door and its thresholds in ways which close it too swiftly, or jam it open too unkindly. We are witnessing the quality of one life being very explicitly defined, judged and ended by another. We share as a society the dilemmas of the proxy agent – doctor, family, carer, court – deciding for the person. These decisions, emotive, and of the utmost sensitivity, are being taken on behalf of others. That is, for those who may not *seem* to have the capacity to decide when others believe a decision is appropriate. The issue here is surely not only that proxy agents may not necessarily decide as the person would decide, if they were able. It is whether *anyone* should have such freedom to intrude on the freedom of another in this way. And, if there are to be any exceptions, on which grounds and with which conscious losses as well as gains. For example, should medically supervised euthanasia be legally available? Should it be open as a choice to the terminally ill, many of whom may dread being kept alive by modern medical technology and who wish to avoid further suffering and, as a final act in life, control their own death? What is the balance to be struck between individual choice, on the one hand, and the social anxiety which suggests that the elderly may be hastened to their deaths and the trust between patients and doctors will be compromised? How might laws be written to preserve that value, permit assisted suicide and absolve clinicians from legal liability – and should they be written at all? There is also the European perspective: will these decisions be made in the UK or in Europe, by an amended European Convention on human rights? And there is the question of how professionals actually behave when presented with a 'living will' and advance directives, whether these are ignored and why.

We may wish to take a high view of motive, to express generous hopes, but the law (in what Hawthorne, discussing 'the moral sillabub', called 'the rust iron framework of society'), must necessarily, too, provide for those circumstances when low motives prevail.

Who is to be in charge and why? If we believe that there is a moral imperative for the proxy agent to so decide, to end suffering, then on what basis of 'knowledge'? On what moral basis? Within which legal framework, within which safeguards, to permit which exceptions? And with which – very likely pervasive – influence on social mores? Even if we wish to advance the risky argument that there should be substituted judgements based on 'knowing what the individual would want', we can agree that much knowledge of others is unknowable, especially in these situations. And the knowledge we do have, for example from disabled people, indicates that many disabled people willingly grasp a quality of life which, for the fully able, seems intolerable. Equally, those who are seriously ill but not otherwise disabled may or may not be willing to accept different levels of pain. Here, the claim is made that someone else knows what is right for you, that they express your 'real' wishes, that they provide you with what you would want if you recognized your 'real' needs, that they know you better than you know yourself.

These are the fundamental questions, which include how to live a good life and a good, dignified death. How to help and guide those in medicine and nursing who seek to help us. How to derive guidance on action, in a moral framework. How to set in place procedures that can be verified in court, and exceptionally to admit mitigating circumstances about the actions of third parties. In considering these questions we need, perhaps above all, a common sense of duty and a requirement of kindness. For this is to be concerned about the care of the disabled but not necessarily convenient; for the pain-racked who do not necessarily wish to be kept alive by an increasingly biotechnical dehumanizing environment (but who should decide?). This is to be concerned, too, for those unable to express a view, but on whom – dutybound – we should wait. And for children, who seem to wish to be the 'main decider' about their treatment, and whose wish and capacity for judgement we seem to have underestimated. Even in an increasingly pluralistic society, we do need a legal system which guides action, one that is based on known if abstract principles and which accommodates the range of cases and dilemmas within a coherent and humane framework. This needs to be rooted in a view of freedom and in an awareness that goals and ideals *are* often conflicting, uncombinable and incommensurable. We need rules that can both be interpreted by the courts and which are sustained by social consent. That is, by a broad agreement about values which we hold in common, either consciously and explicitly, or as we express them by implication in our behaviour, actions and gestures. Those values that we imply in our collective sense of our relations to one another and to our environment, with a cohesive sense of justice and authority, of liberty, of obligation and duty. It is in these areas where people have sought systems and 'rights', but this structure of lighthouses may not now keep us off the rocks.

There seem to me to be at least four different groups of people whose welfare and future arise when we seek to clarify these dilemmas. They cause such terrible and tragic anguish because they focus conflicting values and often uncombinable hopes. Berlin's[3] is the shadow behind the arras. These groups are different, and need to be carefully distinguished. But they share these common philosophical difficulties, notably the question of who is and how to make choices between intolerable alternatives. This makes naked these unavoidable incompatibilities. This asks fundamental questions about the relations of the individual to the community, to the state, to themselves and of each of us to one another. These can only be resolved by selecting imperfect solutions, by personal choice for compromise. Thus, an equilibrium necessarily, if painfully, achieved through toleration and mutual support.

In cases of this kind, the implication of what Berlin says suggests that there can be no principle which tells us how to act. People who acknowledge the same values will make different judgements about freedom, and about trade-offs between liberty and other values. And, forced to choose between virtues that cannot both be achieved, the individual may have to make a decision in the full knowledge that they are renunciating a value which when given up generates an irreparable loss. Here resides the anguish and the human loss. In addition, many may wish to say 'no' to self-knowledge, and to decision-making. 'Autonomy' may be too comprehensive an ideal.

Consider these distinctions, which are matters of knowledge about conflicts of values. They are themselves necessarily pluralistic and contain conflicting elements. This is where these difficulties are actualized, where whatever we do we may commit a wrong, possibly irreparably. For, as Joseph Raz[13] comments: 'Even in success there is a loss, and quite commonly there is no meaning to the judgement that one gains more than one loses'. We are considering here actual people, actual empirical selves, riddled with idiosyncrasy and preference. We should hold tight to the view that this is itself not a bad but a good thing. For these exposed difficulties are necessarily *supported* and *encouraged* by our capacity for choice. And by the pluralist inventiveness and creativity which comes from choice. Computers, too, may allow those 'locked-in' victims who cannot communicate to do so in new and surprising ways.

Consider these distinct categories.

First, those said to be brain-dead and dependent on technology for survival bodily – of whom one such was Tony Bland, the Hillsborough football disaster victim. He was eventually permitted to die, in a proxy decision by the House of Lords on 4 February 1993.[14] He had been in a coma for three years. Obviously, his death was not at his own request, since he was unaware of his condition. It was argued that he was essentially dead, with conscious life irrecoverable. He was said to be dead in life. Medically he was brain-dead. This is a condition Janet Daley[15] has called 'undead'.

Second, those disabled by conditions such as cerebral palsy, and in a vegetative state. These unfortunate patients are like PVS patients, except that they retain their cortex. They are unconscious, but alive. Their lives are not otherwise threatened although they are sustained by dependence on others. This is the case of the extremely unfortunate and afflicted 23 year-old man, known only as 'R', whose case was decided by Sir Stephen Brown, President of the Family Division of the High Court in mid-April 1996.[16-19] Here, was a decision of principle and a quality of life decision. But for a man who was born with very serious disabilities, was conscious, wheelchair bound, who was possibly aware of his condition, who could communicate non-verbally, who could communicate his distress. To whom was his quality of life unacceptable? His family agreed with the South Buckinghamshire NHS Trust that his quality of life was 'unacceptable' to him. The Official Solicitor 'represented' the man, who could not represent himself. (This itself may be thought to be a curious notion.)

Third, those in a deep coma, unconscious and kept alive technologically.

Fourth, those like the 80 year-old liver-cancer patient[20,21] whose son administered a massive morphine overdose to end her excruciating pain and to allow her to die in dignity. This so-called mercy killing which many may feel was a loving act. But there is, of course, the risk of other motives in other cases. This, too, is a proxy judgement unless there is clear prior direction from the sufferer.

Fifth, those who from the beginning of life cannot express themselves, such as young babies. Cases like the profoundly brain-damaged three month-old girl, Baby C[22] of whom a High Court judge recently decided that it was not in the interests of the child to continue to be ventilated artificially. Families face 1000 similar cases each year. Or cases such as the senile elderly or the mentally ill who cannot express themselves, and for whom doctors, nurses, carers make substituted judgements.

Commonly, the issue is posed as the key questions: 'what is an acceptable life? Who is to decide on what is a reasonable definition of an acceptable life? What do we mean by "personhood"?' And how accurate is medicine in assessing internal states of consciousness, quality of life and a balance of benefits and burdens? And in its diagnosis of so-called PVS patients?

What is known as the 'persistent vegetative state' has raised important principles and difficulties. The conceptual language used is open to severe challenge. For each of us should remain a person, irrespective of our situation. We should never be objectified as a thing, a 'vegetable'. Instead, I would prefer to use the expression 'impaired capacity syndrome', which captures the idea that something has happened to someone; some may yet still be re-integrated into society. 'PVS' implies that an individual is no longer a person, yet some few may have those potentials.[a] The situation of such a person takes us back, too, to the fundamental value of autonomy and choice in its influence on the entire society. And to the difficulties of who is to act in the proxy role: doctors, nurses, families, advocates, patient groups, the law? In which circumstances, with which rights, responsibilities and obligations, and to whom? Indeed, we enter, too, the problem of 'rights', which I will skirt here, save to doubt whether all rights (to life?) can be enforced.

The discussion about the persistent vegetative state offers here a very difficult example of the 'best interests' problem, in which others act as proxies. This opens out the basic principles of what kind of society we seek to live

---

[a] Here, the Biomedical and Health Research Programme of the European Commission (BIOMED 1) is seeking clarification in key related areas, including the project on *The Moral and Legal Issues Surrounding the Treatment and Health Care of Patients in Persistent Vegetative State*. This is led by Professor Andrew Grubb of the Centre of Medical Law and Ethics, King's College, London. It aims to identify, clarify and assess the moral principles which are thought to provide the justificatory basis for decisions to withdraw or withhold treatment, through a consideration of the very especial difficulties presented by patients in persistent vegetative state. As the project states: 'For this groups of patients, unlike others for whom the withholding or withdrawing of treatment may sometimes be morally legitimate, are neither brain-dead nor dying, even though they may never regain consciousness and have little prospect of improvement. They therefore raise moral problems of a particularly fundamental kind.' A second project among many concerned with ethical issues is on *Decision-making and Impaired Capacity: The Ethics, Law and Practice Concerning Incompetent Patients*, led by Dr D Evans of the Centre for Philosophy and Health Care, University of Swansea. A third project, on *Ethical Issues in Biomedical Research with Cognitively Impaired Elderly Subjects* is led by Professor RHJ Ter Muelen of the Institute for Bioethics, Maastricht. These projects will need to address the necessarily irreconcilable, the incommensurable, and the fact that as guidelines and European law develop, medical professionals and service users may have the same incentives, but not necessarily so. There is, too, the issue of those situations where treatment is not offered at all, quite aside from when it may be withdrawn in different medical contexts. In September 1996, a BIOMED 2 package was issued by the EC. I owe these references to Professor Andrew Grubb, Director of The Centre of Medical Law and Ethics, King's College, London.

in. We see here, too, an aspect of the rationing difficulty in health care (which, as I argue elsewhere, will be rapidly personalized by the Internet and a multimedia interactive technology in the domestic environment).

The requirement to maintain patient confidentiality and the difficulty of supplying a satisfactory methodology has limited the availability of standardized data on family attitudes and of those of the wider community concerning PVS patients (although we now have some good data on doctors' views – but not yet nurses' – on the 'management' of such patients). We are still limited in our knowledge of both carer and public awareness of the moral issues (and possible ethical clarifications) that arise. Yet informed discussion and consent for legal changes which enshrine practice – for management regimes, and for the protection of patients, medical professionals and carers – is of the essence. We need to develop systematic ways to contact carers and families to involve them in research which will form the basis of practice and policy. To ask such questions as whose expectations are being expressed? How can we evaluate different experiences in different countries, and in different care environments – for example, in the home or in special units? What conclusions can we draw from different experiences and outcomes? There is, too, the further question of who is to consent (and on whose behalf) for what research work. We can go back to fundamentals here: for example, diagnosis and its security is of concern. So, too, is the balance between investment in prevention, treatment and rehabilitation. You and I may think that the emphasis should be on helping people to live, and that we need an emphasis on helping people revive and rehabilitate, and not only on helping people to die. That the effort should be to help to live fuller lives and to improve the speed, location and skills of diagnostic instruments and the information given to families and to the community.

For the PVS, or impaired capacity patient, we confront fundamentals. We need good evidence, and better informed discussion to clarify the moral issues, in order to formulate policy and medical practice. We need to know the experiences of carers especially in this difficult area. This is but one aspect of the persistent and greater need to listen to carers and patients and to speak and act on the basis of the evidence of the stories they have to tell us. How do these decisions relate to an understanding of negative (or positive) freedom and of the separate notion of autonomy? And how do we justify substituted judgements over a parent's or a child's life or death? If we agree on the moral importance of choice, where are the grounds both for direct and, separately, for substituted judgements? Very directly, one might put it thus: 'this is about what is to be done to you, with you, or by you'. And: 'is it up to me, or is it up to you?' The individual is always key if, echoing *As You Like It*, there is to be 'a great reckoning in a little room'.

There is a large philosophical literature concerning the 'right to life', in which many assert this as sacrosanct. They thus deny the choice of self-infliction of death and the involvement of others in carrying out that choice. It has been argued on the one hand that there is an inalienable right to life which underlies the law, and on the other that no new consensus has emerged in society which opposes the right of the state to regulate the involvement of others in exercising power over individuals ending their lives. The natural rights argument avers that human life cannot be deliberately taken away, even with the consent of the individual who loses the life. This has been put less strongly by saying that at the very least the life cannot be taken even with the consent of the person who is to die without independent judicial inquiry or sanction. Clearly, there is a need to protect the weak and vulnerable, to provide judicial sanction and review, to ensure supervision and monitoring, and to protect the presumption of the need to protect and preserve life. The integrity of professionals struggling with these questions is itself an important value to be supported and endorsed.

In the recent Australian debate concerning the right of the terminally ill to end their life it was proposed that they should have the choice of time and manner of death, since seeking to control the manner and timing of one's death constitutes a conscious choice of life over death. Thus, life as a value is engaged even in the case of the terminally ill who themselves seek to choose death over life. In opposition to this view it was argued in principle that this is morally wrong, since there are restraints which even the State has to recognize, and which morally define the State and its role. This case was put powerfully (but unsuccessfully) in an appeal to the Supreme Court of the Northern Territory of Australia. It was also argued that persons terminally ill are particularly vulnerable as to their life and will to live, and that they may not have adequate protection. In this submission it was argued that:

> The plaintiffs say that there are justiciable limits on state action; the submission pre-supposes – pace so-called positivism and realism – that laws are principled and more than mere rules, that there is a sacrosanct value or right any interference with which is illegitimate; it assumes an intrinsic good, unreferable to the wishes of society, and that the state is not the only embodiment of the common good; it asserts something self-evident and underivative such that any legislative interference therewith is wrong; it asserts that such interference is a wrong per se and regardless of the legislation; provenance, ie that the interference is wrong irrespective of whether the 'law' is that of a democratic parliament or a despot; and it asserts that such interference is wrong regardless of its consequences, ie the interference is wrong whether the legislation is otherwise in the public interest or not; the wrong of the legislative interference is not cured by improvising its effects.

Further,

> Implicit in the submission is that individuals have inherent moral status, ie they are an end in themselves – rather than a means to an end – and that treating people as ends in themselves requires more than (or other than) respecting their autonomy.

These are arguments about abstract rights (to liberty, dignity, choice, equality, respect), about morality, about public philosophy, institutional practice, and the moral checks of the law in legislation and case-decisions which we need to address in the wider society, not only in the cloisters of colleges and cathedrals. Clearly, the definition of the problems arises from clear thought and precise language in those properly protected venues about the values which are said to underpin our society. The true nature of these questions is ethical, moral, or political.

The English case of Anthony Bland is of enormous significance, and the judgement of immense value and sophistication. Lord Justice Hoffmann relied on underlying moral principles which he set out in making his legal decision that it was both lawful and right to allow Tony Bland to die in *Airedale NHS Trust v. Bland* (1993) AC 789. He argued that law, morality, and wide social support must coincide. Thus:

> This is not an area in which any difference can be allowed to exist between what is legal and what is morally right. The decision of the court should be able to carry conviction with the ordinary person as being based not merely on legal precedent but also upon acceptable ethical values.

He set out that it is not the function of judges to lay down systems of morals; that there is a strong feeling that there is an intrinsic value in human life, irrespective of whether it is valuable to the person concerned or indeed to anyone else; that these are widely shared intuitive values and – crucially – that 'No law which ignores them can possibly hope to be acceptable'.

Together with the sanctity of life as an ethical principle which we apply to decisions about how we should live there is, too, respect for the individual human being and for his right to choose how to live – individual autonomy, the right of self-determination. Closely connected to this is the principle of respect for the dignity of the individual human being, and the anathema we feel for treating anyone without respect for his value as a human being. Hoffmann, like Berlin, drew attention to the incommensurable. He said: 'No one I think would quarrel with these deeply rooted ethical principles. But what is not always realised, and what is critical in this case, is that they are not always compatible with each other.' Thus, the sanctity of life and the right of self-determination may conflict. A patient may refuse life-saving treatment. Allowing him to choose to die offends the principle of the sanctity of life. Decriminalizing suicide allowed the principle of self-determination to override that of the sanctity of life. It is necessary, Hoffmann argued in the Bland case, to confront these conflicts and to make a choice. Thus:

> A conflict between the principles of the sanctity of life and the individual's right of self-determination may therefore require a painful compromise to be made. In the case of the person who refuses an operation without which he will certainly die, one or other principle must be sacrificed. We may adopt a paternalist view, deny that his autonomy can be allowed to prevail in so extreme a case, and uphold the sanctity of life. Sometimes this looks an attractive solution, but it can have disturbing implications. Do we insist upon patients accepting life-saving treatment which is contrary to their strongly held religious beliefs? Should one force-feed prisoners on hunger strike? English law is, as one would expect, paternalist towards minors. But it upholds the autonomy of adults. A person of full age may refuse treatment for any reason or no reason at all, even if it appears certain that the result will be his death.

Hoffmann is, to my view, right to have stated both that the position taken by English law is not the only morally correct solution but that the fundamental to emphasize is that there is no morally correct solution which can be deduced from a single ethical principle, such as the sanctity of life or self-determination. The complexities which society now confronts require an accommodation between such principles, both of which intuitively seem both rational and good, but which may conflict. It is the accommodation, who is to decide upon it, and how it is to be regulated, which is the debate.

Hoffmann, drawing on a reading of the manuscript of Professor Ronald Dworkin's then forthcoming book *Life's Dominion* (and on conversations with him and with Professor Bernard Williams), brilliantly clarified the conflicting and prismatic ethical principles in the Bland case. For Anthony Bland was alive, and the principle of the sanctity of life said that he should not deliberately be allowed to die. Yet he was a human being who, on the principle of self-determination, should be allowed to choose for himself. By definition and problematically, however, in his case, he was unable to express his choice and had no prospect of recovery. Hoffmann stated:

> If he is unable to express his choice, we should try our honest best to do what we think he would have chosen. We cannot disclaim this choice because to go on is as much a choice as to stop.

Hoffmann added:

> Normally we would unquestionably assume that anyone would wish to live rather than to die. But in the extraordinary case of Anthony Bland, we think it more likely that he would choose to put an end to the humiliation of his being and the distress of his family. Finally, Anthony Bland is a person to whom respect is owed and we think that it would show greater respect to allow him to die and be mourned by his family than to keep him grotesquely alive.

The anguish arises because we have no formulae to which we can appeal by which we can reconcile this conflict of principles. This is the territory of Berlin's incommensurables with which we began. As Hoffmann said:

> It does no good to seize hold [of one principle], such as the sanctity of life, and say that because it is valid and right, as it undoubtedly is, it must always prevail over other principles which are also valid and right. Nor do I think it helps to say that these principles are all really different ways of looking at the same thing. Counsel appearing as amicus said that there was 'no inherent conflict between having regard to the quality of life and respecting the sanctity of life; on the contrary they are complementary; the principle of sanctity of life embraces the needs for full respect to be accorded to the dignity and memory of the individual'.

I stand with Hoffmann (and surely Berlin) here when he says: 'To my mind, this is rhetoric intended to dull the pain of having to choose'. Hoffmann himself then cited Berlin's *Two Concepts of Liberty*[23] to codify the situation we face:

> The world that we encounter in ordinary experience is one in which we are faced with choices between ends equally ultimate, and claims equally absolute, the realisation of some of which must inevitably involve the sacrifice of others ... The knowledge that it is not merely in practice but in principle impossible to reach clear-cut and certain answers, even in an ideal world of wholly good and rational men and wholly clear ideas, may madden those who seek for final solutions and single, all-embracing systems, guaranteed to be eternal. Nevertheless, it is a conclusion that cannot be escaped by those who, with Kant, have learnt the truth that out of the crooked timber of humanity no straight thing was ever made.

Values collide. All good things cannot be harmonized in principle. Particular virtues may not be able to be maximized, save by diminishing other virtues. Berlin has unequivocally and disturbingly advised us of the pluralist possibility (which may be no comfort to many) that 'there are many different ends that men may seek and still be fully rational, fully men, capable of understanding each other and sympathising and deriving light from each other'. And:

> The notion of the perfect whole, the ultimate solution, in which all good things coexist, seems to me to be not merely unattainable – that is a truism – but conceptually incoherent; I do not know what is meant by a harmony of this kind. Some among the Great Goods cannot live together. That is a conceptual truth. We are doomed to choose, and every choice must entail an irreparable loss. Happy are those who live under a discipline which they accept without question, who freely obey the orders of leaders, spiritual or temporal, whose word is fully accepted as unbreakable law; or those who have, by their own methods, arrived at clear and unshakeable convictions about what to do and what to be that brook no possible doubt. I can only say that those who rest on such comfortable beds of dogma are victims of forms of self-induced myopia, blinkers that may make for contentment, but not for understanding of what it is to be human.

Lord Justice Hoffmann emphasized that law cannot evade the responsibility for decision, but that it must be embedded in wider intuitions. Thus:

> In my view the choice which the law makes must reassure people that the courts do have full respect for life, but that they do not pursue the principle to the point at which it becomes almost empty of any real content and when it involves the sacrifice of other important values such as human dignity and freedom of choice.

The difficulty of 'substituted judgements', of course, remains, when we ask how can we 'know' another human being (let alone 'know' ourselves), and how can we 'know' what we think Anthony Bland would have chosen? The grounds, values, morality and social sanction for such judgements, together with the legal process, needs to be stated with arctic clarity and managed with the utmost dignity, honesty, and sensitivity.

These issues are, of course, historically and culturally specific, and that is commonly said. But the general principle of valuing choice can be argued as a consistent element. Observably, of course, responsible professionals, caring parents and families, and individuals considering their own fate, may behave differently in different cultures. In the USA two federal appeal courts have recently upheld the right of terminally ill people to commit suicide with the help of a doctor. This issue now seems likely to go to the US Supreme Court where justices will be asked to decide if the dying have a constitutional right to ask a doctor for assistance in ending their lives. The American Medical Association has decided to review its objections. In the USA the problem is known as 'the immortality ethic'. There, these issues are fought around the concept of civil rights. The federal appeal court voted eight to three recently that competent adults have a constitutional right to seek help in choosing 'a dignified and humane death rather than being reduced to a child-like state of helplessness'. A similar finding followed in New York. Current UK cases make explicit that our attempts at elaboration of the relationship between ethical principles and actions have not yet provided definitive guidelines. Yet medical professionals, the patients, carers and families, have to make often emotive decisions daily. Here, our only certainty may be uncertainty until we can agree rules which accommodate a range of options, rooted in clarity about what we mean by choice. Uncertainty, however, is not a sustainable policy.

Existing approaches to 'living wills' (advance directives), for example, are a genuine beginning. But these seem too unspecific, and, in their necessary interpretation, too reliant on professional judgements. Few now make them, although there is guidance on samples and there are those willing to give guidance. Many people, of course, do not make even an ordinary will, despite wide knowledge of them. Living and ordinary wills do, too, necessarily, 'date'. Advance directives do not have clear legal status, in spite of accumulating case law. Many professionals – for example, the Royal College of Nursing and the Terrence Higgins Trust – have thought very sensitively about these issues. There are, here, contingent discussions about the personal responsibility of all actors, and the true source of 'responsibility' – about myth and mystique in medicine, about uncertainty and how to confess it, about new technology and new information. About the end of masonic information and the redesign of intelligence for the consumer. About incentive and sanction, selection, education and socialization.

My topic is existential. My general conclusion is that we need to think through again our existing cultural frameworks, which emphasize controls. We need to review our medical model, our disease and health care model, what patients can and should contribute, in terms of a reiterated belief in the personal and cultural importance of choice. And we should also reconsider the determinants of health care which we may or may not be able to influence, but which may tell us something important about self-esteem, choice and empowerment. My method, please forgive, is both philosophic and poetic, for this is about feelings and values as much as about p's and q's. My specific conclusion is that I take choice and thus empowerment, to be *the* outcome.

In this discussion I consider some dilemmas in two principle areas: first, those concerned with who is to decide about the quality of a life; and, second, the general question of how health service users can be empowered.

In considering how to consider these issues, I looked for solace and comfort to the poet Walt Whitman. His is surely wise, if implied, advice. Be allusive, not merely didactic. That is, don't let the chalk squeak. For he writes:

> Tell all the truth but tell it slant.
> Success in circuit lies
> Too bright for our inform Delight
> The truth's superb surprise.

Let us enquire within of the truth's superb surprise. Its light is often too bright.

Where is my country?

Public solace in medicine is often sought where it is embedded culturally – in myth and mystique. This is one part of the inherited geology of culture. It is one of the fundamental constraints which obstruct choice, with all the damaging disadvantages which flow from that barrier. It is both an internal and then an externalized constraint which helps prevent the individual from perceiving alternatives as such. It hinders action even when alternatives are perceived. It is sabotage from within. It is in this restriction of choice – the limits on 'negative' freedom – that the most fundamental 'un-freedoms' are to be found. Thus, 'myth and mystique' is as incapacitating as the absence of knowledge, money and other resources which themselves impair the capacity of the individual to act in freedom, for choice, for personal resolution of moral dilemmas and for better health care.

Here, I am reminded of a story John Keane reports in his biography of Tom Paine[24]: 'Where liberty is, there is my country', Benjamin Franklin once reportedly remarked to Tom Paine. 'Where liberty is not, there is my country', Paine replied. Who owns our bodies? I am uneasy that the answer is too often envisaged in the controls of a cultural system and by an élite minority of which both Paine and William Blake warned England more than a century ago. One which disempowers the individual and validates the veto of special interests. That is, who controls what, and for which purposes within a framework of general ethical rules rigorously derived and analysed, and which discipline practice. We need to decide this on the basis, too, of wide, democratic debate. And with plain-language guidance. For, as John Keane reminds us, 'words are deeds ... liberty is connected with prose ... [and] people unfriendly to citizens' liberty normally wrap their power in pompous or meaningless phrases.' 'Bastilles of the word' was Paine's phrase for this error.

We need, too, a structure of compelling devices which genuinely empower the individual for the unexpected, which they derive from within themselves.

We need, too, an open approach to these complexities which does not of itself close out the ordinary. It will be evident that there are few more difficult cultural tasks. And there are perhaps no more obtuse countries. For, as Neil Belton[25] has recently stated succinctly: 'English culture is full of antiquated barricades, tollgates at crossing points between forms of imagination that should be free and open.' Is this not, particularly in medicine, an example of what the anthropologist Clifford Geertz[26] meant when he wrote of closed societies, in which he saw 'The sense of intellectual self-sufficiency, that peculiar conceptual and methodological arrogance which comes from dealing too long and too insistently with a pocket universe all one's own'?

Medical mystery is one barricade. Another is the emphasis on health care and disease as the chief determinant of health status. A third is the political market, with its reliance on unelected, powerful, brokering and mediating veto-organizations. These sustain a mismatch between the possibility and the fact of choice, between a modern, mass-consumer society energized by informed choice and a society structured and powerfully managed by an élite in a political market. The impact of official structures of medicine, one of the cultural foundations (and political instruments) of the state, is a principal characteristic of what the economist James Buchanan called public-choice theory, or the politics of the market.[27–29] Here, votes count as much as patients. All of this impacts on the deepest nature of our society, and on our individual potential to face moral dilemmas. It impacts, especially, on our capacity for self-management in modern health care.

We must ensure, too, that this debate is not only about medicine and disease, about what John Stuart Collis – adjusting Burton – called 'the melancholy of anatomy', but about cultures and communities, about how we live together now. For the query as to who owns our bodies is an issue both about the fundamentals of personal identity, and of what really determines health (however that is to be defined). It concerns what the wider culture endorses in its politics and its attitudes. This is to notice, but not *en passant*, several essential questions about the NHS. This is to look at the question of the performance of the NHS as a health care system in cultural terms, not least the impact of its predominant attitudes and behaviours on the quality of individual, self-reflective lives and on the wider economic success or failure of the nation. These are the pivotal, defining, cultural processes of permanent possession through dispossession which characterize NHS power relations in a political marketplace. It is political will, not patient incapacity, which is restricting patient choice and empowerment.

Here, it is my submission that any difficulties of running the system on the basis of individual choice are not organizational. They are a matter of point of view and of power. It is politics which maroons the fly in the bottle. It is politics which is preventing empowerment from becoming a country instead of simply a distant coastline.

We should keep reminding ourselves that these matters of the situations individuals, families and carers confront, are not only matters for the academy, or for policy analysts. These issues are about real people. People in sometimes terrible excruciating pain, about real human loss and grief, about bereavement of husbands from wives, mothers from children, about terrible moral and practical dilemmas. About decisions like cutting off life support for those unable to speak, hear, see, or 'know', whom one loves very deeply. There is no clear framework. But these things do not only happen in the cinema; they are racking real people every day. They require practical thought about how to help people help themselves.

The Daily Mail[30] on 18 April 1996, and *The Daily Telegraph*[31] on 19 April 1996, reported on *The Rights of the Terminally Ill Act*, passed by the government of the Northern Territory, Australia. This Act may well presage the way forward in many countries for patients wishing to assert the right to control his or her own death in some circumstances. It became law on 1 July 1996. The Act enables patients to avail themselves of voluntary euthanasia – and thus to assert their independence and their wish to be in control at the end. The Act stipulates that a patient, who must be at least 18 years of age and experiencing pain, suffering or distress to an extent unacceptable to him or her, may ask a doctor for help to die. The key is a new computer-screen system, with a program entitled 'Deliverance', which the patient can control even when in extreme pain and because they wish to die, exercising their autonomy. The program uses an adaptation of Microsoft Access, a database program that runs on Windows PCs.

The Rights of the Terminally Ill Act 1995 (Northern Territory) establishes a regulatory framework for the intentional termination of human life in stipulated circumstances. It does so within the Australian Constitution (which embodies fundamental values) whilst removing all criminal, civil and professional sanctions which are otherwise applicable to a medical practitioner who intentionally terminates a patient's life or assists a patient to commit suicide. As it was stated during the Australian debate, the Act may fundamentally change the medical profession's norm, and not merely regulate it in a new way. For:

> The Act institutionalises intentional killing which would otherwise be murder; it institutionalises aiding suicide which would otherwise be a crime.

The preamble of the Act provides that it is:

> An Act to confirm the right of a terminally ill person to request assistance from a medically qualified person to voluntarily terminate his or her life in a humane manner; to allow for such assistance to be given in certain circumstances without legal

impediment to the person rendering the assistance; to provide procedural protection against the possibility of abuse of the rights recognised by this Act; and for related purposes.

'Terminal illness' is carefully defined, as is the framework within which each party must behave.

There is a 22-step process with many clear safeguards. A number of doctors must be involved and there are fail-safe and 'cooling-off' stipulations for the patient's decision-making process. Two doctors with at least five years medical experience each must be involved, one with a diploma in psychiatry. Each must have diagnosed the patient as terminally ill and beyond medical help. First, a doctor, who must be from the Northern Territory, has to be satisfied that the patient has a fatal illness which has no chance of a cure. A second doctor with experience in the illness, must agree with the first assessment. This doctor who must be a psychiatrist, has to confirm that the patient is not suffering from 'a treatable clinical depression'. The patient must be informed of all palliative care options. At least seven days after the first request from the patient the individual may request a formal document, the 'Request for Assistance to End My Life in a Humane and Dignified Manner'. There must then be a further 48 hour cooling-off period. Doctors will be required to witness the patient signing. The patient must then wait for a further 48 hours for the requested administration of lethal drugs. This administration of drugs must be carried out in the presence of the first doctor. It is reported that a Dr Philip Nitschke, together with a computer expert, had developed a euthanasia device which enables the individual to express their decision by keying into a computer. The computer screen is reported to offer options, including: 'If you press "YES", you will cause a lethal injection to be given within 30 seconds and will die. Do you wish to proceed?' Then: 'Are you certain that you understand that if you proceed and press the "YES" button on the next screen that you will die? "YES/NO"'. Then: 'In 15 seconds you will be given a lethal injection ... "YES/NO"'. Then a syringe will drip lethal drugs into the patient's arm. The patient will fall asleep and will then die in minutes.

Mrs Jan Culhane, a terminally ill nurse, is reported by *The Daily Mail*[30] as saying: 'I'm by no means in more pain than I've ever seen people survive under, but it's pain that I'm not willing to accept. What is non-acceptable to me is probably acceptable to somebody else.'[a]

Should we adopt such a system, celebrating autonomy?

---

[a] The first patient to end his life by legally sanctioned euthanasia in Australia was Mr Ben Dent, a 66 year-old cancer sufferer, on 22 September 1996. See Celia Hall, 'Disagree with voluntary euthanasia ... but don't deny the right to me', *The Daily Telegraph*, 27 September 1996. The law came into force on 1 July 1996.

Cont'd

The big sky

There are here several big-sky issues. Let me pick two.

First, ideological: what kind of a society do we want to live in, what is the acceptable structure of liberty for both the individual and the encapsulating community? Here, again, is self-creation, self-transformation and choice. Second, practical: what can we expect from a disease-focused health care system and what other action is necessary to influence health status? What are the determinants of health, how can these be influenced? Most especially, what do they tell us about the impact on health of self-reflection and self-esteem, as a hint of the alchemical yield of wider empowerment in 'negative' liberty? Here, I call in the aid of a health economist, Robert G Evans[32] (recommended to me by another, Tony Cullyer). I do so as a prelude to my coming argument about the wider potential of 'empowerment' of the patient and service user, which will remit our deficits and engage all values.

First, it looks as if the impact of self-esteem and empowerment is much underestimated. It looks as if this is a vital sign, possibly carried through into impact on immune systems. It looks as if the medical model and its impact on disease is overestimated as a source of health status. I offer this idea, which I derive from Evans[32] and from McKeown's[33] work showing that environmental and not medical influences were the principal source of dramatic reductions in disease and deaths in England and Wales. The American work by the McKinleys[34] argues such a case, too.

Evans suggests[32] that change may well need to be about that elusive item, self-esteem. And that patient empowerment, together with the wider empowerment and the personal esteem derived by the individual in every socio-economic class from the success of the wider society, is the philosopher's stone, the source of alchemy, the pivot of improved mortality and morbidity for populations. This does not let anyone off of the hook of having to make difficult moral and ethical judgements, of course, nor of supporting the demands of long-term chronic care. But it may be the answer to empowerment in other key areas. Leonard A Sagan[35] has argued that there is some general factor or factors about modern society which has made people more resilient and self-confident. Edward Tenner[36] has more recently added this gloss: 'Many disease microorganisms are present in individuals who never develop symptoms; differences in immune response

---

Plaintiffs applied to The Supreme Court of the Northern Territory of Australia to prevent the implementation of *The Rights of the Terminally Ill Act 1995 (Northern Territory)*. The discussion offers an important commentary on the philosophical issues involved, including the nature of rights and the challenges of conflicting goods, on which I have drawn here. See *CJ Wake and D Gondarra vs Northern Territory of Australia and the Hon. KJ Austin, AC, QC, the Administrator of the Northern Territory of Australia, Supreme Court of the Northern Territory of Australia*, 112, 1996, judgement delivered on 24 July, 1996.

must be the cause. Those who feel in control of their future apparently have stronger immune systems ... Conversely, poverty seems to engender a self-destructive fatalism.' Scottish experience is eloquent here.

Tenner[36] writes:

> We are left with an uncomfortable conclusion about health, and especially about longevity. For all the contributions of medical technology, other things have meant more. The real mechanisms of improved health are so entangled in other good things – the economy, education, environmental quality – that we still don't understand just what has happened. We know, as Aaron Wildavsky put it so well, that richer is better. But because we don't understand how and why, it is difficult rationally to say exactly what sorts of public and private applications of money will do most for health. The statistics don't necessarily imply that funds should be shifted from medicine to education, though they may suggest that raiding education programs to pay for health care may have unexpected revenge effects on health itself. Good health turns out to be a positive by-product of the pursuit of other things.

It looks as if self-esteem may be vital in the framework for improved health status. It may be very important in enabling us to live a good life and to die one, too. The impact of empowerment, of control over our own bodies, of the engagement of our values and coping strategies about today and the future warrants attention. Here, perhaps, is another important reason for the due (overdue?) modesty of health care systems, of providers and of professionals.

Researchers ask: 'Why do top people live longer and generally healthier lives?' Many studies in many countries have shown over many years a correlation between life expectancy and various measures of social status – income, education, occupation, residence and health status, which looks to be correlated with social status. But this observation, commonplace now, raises complex questions about the determinants of health, for both individuals and 'populations'. To my mind it raises issues of empowerment.

Evans[32] argues that many conventional explanations about why some people are healthier than others are incomplete or even wrong. Yet massive investment goes into health care systems, the argument being that the reception of appropriate health care – whatever that is, whoever decides that, with what hardly checked results – is the most important determinant of health. However, if the principal determinants of the health of populations lie elsewhere, we may well have, as Evans puts it, 'left undone those things that we ought to have done, and have done those things that we ought not to have done'.

Expanding preventative activities will not necessarily help if our assumptions about the determinants of health are inadequate. 'Curative' services may be the wrong over-emphasis, too, though we need them to relieve suffering. Certainly, the availability of such services, or their absence, does not seem to explain observed differences among the health of populations. So, what is it that we need to look at to establish a more complex, more comprehensive, coherent understanding of the determinants of health?

There seems to be a strong relationship between hierarchy and health and its effects are large. There seems to be some underlying general causal process correlated with hierarchy which *expresses* itself through different diseases. These different diseases may simply be alternative pathways, however, rather than causes of illness and death. That is, they may be the mechanisms through which another essential factor is expressed. So, the idea of looking at the gradient of mortality between social classes and the idea of diseases as pathway, rather than cause of, differential mortality by socioeconomic class warrant careful study. As Evans[32] says: 'While death is ultimately quite democratic, deferral appears to be a privilege correlated with rank.' There is something very striking here. Indices over decades show that even though the causes of death have changed, the mortality gradient persists. This suggests that there is an underlying factor, correlated with hierarchy and expressing itself through particular diseases.

The longitudinal data from the UK show no evidence that the introduction of the NHS has reduced the mortality gradient. So whatever it is that underlies the gradient does not seem to respond to the provision of health care. And note that the very large reductions in mortality from the principal infectious diseases which have occurred over the last two centuries took place prior to the development of any effective medical therapy. For example, tuberculosis. Mortality decline (as McKeown[33] shows and the McKinleys[34] echo) pre-dated therapy. Care did have an impact later – but the limited later role of medicine was swamped by the much larger impact of something else operating outside the health care system. It is this initiating force that we want to understand. And to build on, if we can. McKeown found very large changes in mortality in a society over time; Marmot[37] and others found large differences among social groups over short periods of time. And in these cases these mortality changes seem independent of medical knowledge or care use. So economists ask, 'What are the causal factors that are correlated with hierarchy – status, empowerment, stress, coping skills, future orientation, other factors – and can they be changed?'.

Why do I go into this at length? My purpose is to lead us to empowerment. To heightened personal choice. Evans[37] and his colleagues ask: 'What is it that produces the biological processes that the data reports?' As Evans says: 'While people always die of something – this is both a cultural convention and a requirement of modern systems of vital statistics – there is reason to believe that the particular diseases recognised by medical science may not be the fundamental causes'. What Evans says of Japan seems to me to be especially persuasive. There, the health status of an entire population has changed very rapidly. Why?

Since 1960 Japanese mortality statistics (male and female life expectancy and infant mortality) have improved from markedly below most European countries to markedly above and the trend may be continuing. Why has there been an extraordinary increase in Japanese life expectancy? It does not appear to follow from better medical care. Japan has not expanded health care investment more than most. The environment generally is not a healthy one. Nor does the explanation look like diet or social structure; indeed, changes here would seem unhelpful rather than helpful. In any case, they have not been rapid over a long-run of 30 years.

However, Evans[37] suggests that what *has* changed is the hierarchical position of Japanese society as a whole, relative to the rest of the world. Clearly, being Japanese has been a better way to feel about oneself in some important sense. If you like, this is an academic way of saying you are healthier when you are having fun.

It looks as if large macro-environmental factors, both social and physical, may have an extremely large influence on illness patterns. It is evident, too, that what were thought to be nearly fixed boundaries are very moveable, that disease patterns and health status can change rapidly and by a large amount when external factors change. This is a complex area of study, but it does look as if there is something special about success in coping with one's environment and a strong correlation between personal health and the external esteem of a whole society which influences self-esteem. There seem to be health status results of self-esteem, and, it seems to me, of feelings of empowerment. We are only now beginning to understand the way in which these influences exert themselves in biological channels. We are, too, opening out the view that there is much more to being healthy than simply being alive, which is an important insight in clarifying and addressing the quandaries of who owns our bodies.

Our apparently fixed measures of health status, as Tom Paine might have said, look conceptually dodgy. They look malleable, too, in terms of individual values. Self-actualization and self-esteem seem to matter a lot, although we do not know how low self-esteem kills you, if it does, and if that is the unknown which prompts what Evans calls 'the disease as expression'.

How we are to create the conditions for well-lived lives, at a time of unprecedented technical and social external change, is another conundrum. Personally, my prejudice is for liberty.

What of the NHS? Let me turn to that. The individual seeks two things from the NHS: epic and intimate. Epic is the comfort and reassurance of knowing that guaranteed service is there when wanted. Intimate is individual, specific, relevant, timely, quality care which delivers both survival and quality of life on terms and in terms of individual values. Yet health status is primarily determined elsewhere. And the health care system is presently one of controls in a political market place. So, perhaps, instead, we do need to look very carefully at the greater framework of liberty, at sources of self-esteem and notably at education. If the key to a good society and to improving health status is an emphasis on the primacy of the individual, in a minimal or limited state. With the maximum possible personal choice and the maximum encouragement for self-esteem. It is this which will enable optimal care and strengthened community: being easy and free without being free and easy, as well as helping self-management in modern community health care. In such a society achievement, choice and fellowship ought *all* to be achievable. The will to succeed and the wish to assist, the attitudes and behaviours of individual liberty and wider fulfilment, mutually re-inforcing. And, to give this an Asian accent, egalitarian courage in the face of failure will not support a Britain which must set sail for southern continents.

Here, more notably than any other area of human society, we need to hear and consider the cultural barriers noticed by William Faulkner, who says in *Requiem for a nun*[38]: 'The past is never dead; it's not even past.'

This is all to argue that it is ideas which embody a commanding view of what medicine, government and politics might be or are to be about. This poses the question of what is knowledge – about health status, about what it is to speak of health and its determinants and about what is relevant knowledge? How does each kind of knowledge – rationalist, scientific and personal, existential, as well as clinical and socio-economic – impact on what we say is good and not good health, and on practice. And, 'en passant, if suspicion begins at home, what is it that is so special about the values of patients and what so suspicious, by the by, about the renewed emphasis on evidence-based care? For here there is some suspicion that doctors will give up an emphasis on individual autonomy if they can sustain collective autonomy. Whose evidence, too? To what purpose? Is the emphasis on evidence-based care, which offers some technical gains, a call to 'leave it to us' – the doctors – and then all will be well again? John Hersey,[39] in his philosophical angling book, *Blues*, mentions that he keeps 'having this image of the fisherman being caught by the fish, instead of the other way around'. And, further on, 'It all comes down to wanting to *see* – to penetrate the mirror and not just see one's self and one's world'. Or, stated directly, this discussion is about how we set (and could change) the limits and significance of patients in how we (or they) run things. Changing what Paul Carter[40] in a different context has called, 'The glare of an uninterruptedly symmetrical horizon [which has] blindfolded the explorer'.

'A' for autonomy?

Who owns our bodies? The key to all this is choice. And, despite the limitations Berlin[3] notices, the notion of autonomy also matters. But this key may not fit all doors.

We need a beginning, nevertheless. Immanuel Kant[41] wrote helpfully of autonomy and slipped its leash. Kant defined autonomy as moral freedom, which he proposed as the vital element in our moral identity. Mill set this in a social and political context of behaviour, proposing that individual liberty, personal autonomy, was essential to our development and happiness, and thus good for society as a whole.

For Mill the individual was 'the person most interested in his own well-being'.

More recently the ethical philosopher Erich Loewy[42] has put it thus: 'Knowing that we are "the captains of our fate", rather than surmising that we are the pawns of another (no matter how benevolent that other might be), is what most adults, at least in Western culture, want'. In the exercise of this captaincy, the bio-medical good is not the only value that the patient will consider in a hierarchy of personal goods. But does the principle of respect for individual patient autonomy necessarily and always serve as a comfortable guide to action?

Let me consider some contexts, some circumstances where discussion arises of whether or not to prolong life or allow death. For vulnerable infants and for some of the elderly this is especially problematic and emotive. For they lack the capacity to request that treatment be withheld or withdrawn. They often depend on proxy decision-makers. With infants there is no 'substituted judgement' which can be rendered, as their present and past values are unknowable. But the adult individual will perhaps increasingly seek to exercise a choice in advance with regard to aggressive medicine (much of it seemingly futile, costly, and unproductively painful). Resuscitation denied, or insisted upon. Life-prolonging treatment accepted and welcomed, or imposed. An advance agreement, carefully considered with counselling and advice, within the law, signed and available, or a best guess. Notice, too, that there are doctors who appear to believe that death is optional. Equally, we now know that severely handicapped people make different judgements from non-handicapped people about quality of life; that they can find a quality of life rewarding which the unhandicapped may find intolerable. Are these areas where only doctors can decide?

Here, it is argued by some, even loving parents can make choices, perhaps on religious grounds, which conflict with the child's interests, and the doctor may need to intervene as the child's advocate even if this is to end treatment and therefore to end life.

This is very difficult terrain. Consider, for example, the case reported in *The Times*, 13 April 1996,[21] of the caring and loving son whose 80 year-old mother, Alice Rowbottom, was reported as unable to eat, drink, move or speak without crying. She was dying of liver cancer. Her son Derek is said to have been unable to tolerate leaving her in agony, and to have interfered with the hospital diamorphine pump to administer a massive intravenous dose. His wife subsequently said she would want him to do the same for her in a similar situation. We do not know if his mother had expressed such a wish, and if so, in which mental state, under which conditions and on which terms. For each of us these issues are special, yet some cannot speak for themselves. They may nevertheless remind us of what one reviewer said of a novel by Paul Theroux: 'This is Paul Theroux's journey around himself'. But with which maps? Where is the Captain Cook in this new-met ocean?

This is not about facts, but about values. This is not only a struggle about the status of medical technique, or about the Enlightenment and its rationale of scientific explanation. Indeed, the Counter-Enlightenment view that science and reason do not have all the answers has endorsed the notion that the central ethical, aesthetic and social questions of value can have several valid answers. The struggle is existentialist. It is about emotion and feeling, as a fulcrum for committed, informed choice. It is not about the reduction of the complex to the simple. Rather, it consists, as Levi-Strauss says, 'in the substitution of a complexity more intelligible for one which is less'.

It is, too, a simultaneous ambition to humanize dehumanizing social institutions and to create an environment in which medical professionals and patients can work most successfully together. This is not – as I will argue momentarily – the same thing at all as that which the NHS wants to term 'partnership'. For that is an analogue for renewed control in a political market place.

The assumption of self-responsibility for one's actions is a principal characteristic of being human and is of the essence of morality. And, as the ethicist Soren Holm[43] says, 'advice is only advice if it can be rejected. If there is a duty to collaborate with the doctor, then it must be understood as a duty to collaborate in the diagnostic process until sufficient information has been gathered to make a treatment decision, at which point the patient is free to make his own decision'.

Let us look at some of the cases that come up. Consider our new technological medicine, which is enabling us to have more knowledge, more power; over nature, over the human body, over disease, over other people, or over ourselves. This poses huge questions: Is all human life to be treated as sacred? Are all lives to be maintained to the utmost, and irrespective of cost? Are all health investment demands to take priority over other social investments?

Consider that society as a whole fosters an interventionist rather than a preventative approach to disease and often thwarts at any cost (and at the price sometimes of excruciating pain and 'side-effects') what can be the natural course of life. Consider the impact on our social and economic structures and on our health, of unconsidered and rapacious new technologies, which have a comprehensive impact but are evaluated philosophically and practically but only *post hoc*. These have the power to do great good and great harm. Consider dilemmas of social choice. Should everyone have the right to produce a child of their own genetic heritage and should the economic costs be borne by the tax payer? Or the possibilities of genetic engineering and the intrusions of potential abortion expanding as screening expands knowledge prior to birth. In addition, what are children capable and incapable of deciding about their own health care? Do we underestimate their capability to make major personal decisions?

Consider such acknowledged dilemmas as the illegitimacy of self-harm of the proposed suicide. Or another problem of substituted judgement, that of 'helping' the mentally challenged, instead of aiding them to achieve goals they set for themselves as a way of exerting influence and control over their lives and changing everyday feelings of powerlessness. Here, we need to make a beginning at the beginning. We need the empowered involvement of users in helping professionals to see in new ways.

Consider the perplexities with the infant born with major congenital abnormalities, particularly of the central nervous system. The child whose brain has been damaged by infection, haemorrhage, or by hypoxic-ischaemic encephalopathy, the baby with spinida bifida or Down's syndrome, the dependent child or relative whose carer is a Jehovah's Witness. Are these treatment decisions about the quality of life of the child, or of someone else?

Consider, too, the externally unmeasurable – what Gavin Fairbairn[44] called 'the slippery concept', the personal evaluation of 'quality of life', which others seek to judge.

Consider the patient, mentally competent, insisting on the right to decide to end his own life. An argument based on the moral requirement that people respect another's autonomy. And consider the autonomy of the doctor – also, of course, a moral agent – refusing to discharge the patient who will die in the community if untended, and who may yet want to make this choice as a patient.

Consider the patient in the Bolam case.[45] In Britain the law says that if enough doctors are providing a certain treatment – such as long-term diazepam for depression – then the treatment becomes that of a 'reasonably competent practitioner'. That is, in law if enough doctors do it, then it is right. What this means is that even *outside* medicine, there is not one official implement in place to insist that doctors critically assess, perpetually, what they are doing. The patient who wants to hit back with the autonomy stick is in a fix.

Consider, as does Loewy,[42] the suggestion that doctors do not always warn of likely disaster ahead with specific treatments, or that persons are sometimes forced to undergo interventions which those forcing the intervention would reject for themselves. This is becoming an open book at the end of life. It has been repeatedly shown that most patients are aware of their own imminent death, yet many are being kept alive against the wishes of the individual and the family and are denied involvement in such a decision. This emasculates them and reduces their standing in the community, as well as inducing fear. Consider that this converts what should be a humanizing, a nurturing environment into one perceived or feared to be threatening. This is a challenge to the ultimate comfort of the dying.

Consider in which circumstances and how we could pass power to doctors to make decisions on our behalf. Consider the problems of whether or not doctors can with any degree of accuracy know what their patients may want. Research has shown them to be in error. Consider doctors inevitably shrouding value judgements in technical justifications; doing good by breaching autonomy, or refusing to deliver an ineffective treatment. Further, that patients can make choices which fail to express their autonomy or which doctors or nurses may judge damage them, being based on 'mistaken' judgements of value.

All of this discussion is inevitably, but properly, value-laden. These are the acknowledged problems in considering the limitations to autonomy and the principle of respect for others. Insanity, immaturity, senility and the potential to cause oneself harm, the potential constraints of mental incompetence and ignorance, all offer the diminished status which may allow autonomy to be overruled. On what basis? Each prompts, to my mind, wariness and suspicion of paternalistic action. Do we have to decide between strong (that is, insistent) and weak (that, is advisory) paternalism and appropriateness – whatever that word indicates as a kind of knowledge? Or is a simpler commitment to 'choice' not a more satisfactory solution? There are those radically opposed to either. Others make no attempt to defend medical paternalism, nor medical domination of interactions with patients, or even the duty to perform medically indicated treatments as the rationale for overriding respect for individual autonomy. Some ethicists, whilst not discussing choice as a different notion to autonomy, doubt the validity of the physician imposing their judgement even to maximize the autonomy of the patient.

Of course, the notion that doctors ought to make judgements of what is best for patients depends on arguable assumptions, of which the most important is that doctors know what is likely to be medically best. Further, that doctors practise best-practice, with generally equivalent skills more or less, that they respond to research knowledge, that medicine as a body of knowledge is generally certain and that they keep up to date. There is a significant body of research that says otherwise. Further, that many doctor–patient encounters are those of expertise meeting with ignorance, whereas they are two value systems meeting. Even so, *someone* has to take responsibility in many difficult situations and it is often doctors and nurses, often asked by families and carers, who do.

There are many other problems. The fact that an informed patient makes an informed choice does not imply necessarily that that choice reflects what he values. Further, such decisions can harm the functioning of doctors as moral agents which requires them to make evaluations of what patients ought to do, all things considered.

Julian Savulescu,[46] the Oxford philosopher, makes the case for what he calls 'rational non-interventional paternalism'. This is a practice in which doctors form conceptions of what is best for their patients and argue rationally with them, without quite being committed to doing what doctor thinks best. He does rely on the imperative that doctors ought to make judgements, but asks should they be able to insist and to compel? Savulescu argues that medicine must have a commitment to values and not merely to consumerism. And that these values would and must more helpfully direct standards of care than mass consumer choice – which can be irrational, chaotic, apathetic and ill-suited to provide direction alone. Equally, he suggests that informed public opinion should guide practice, that informed discussion and argument can help patients make better decisions for themselves. The values of the profession should, he argues, be more substantial than a commitment to do what every individual patient desires.

In making decisions to do serious things to patients, it is not clear that doctors can avoid making value judgements, or can avoid directional advice. These can be difficult to spot, as Savulescu notes. It depends on how the advice is framed, the manner in which information is presented and how non-verbal clues function. When choice is framed in terms of gain, we are risk-taking; when it is framed in terms of loss, we are risk-averse. For example, the attractions of surgery are greatest when framed in terms of the probability of living rather than the probability of dying.

Shared decision-making seems to some to offer a way through the maze. This offers a movement away from paternalism, so that facts other than medical 'facts' influence action. This engages the individual's values in determining what is best. Each participant seeks to form a best judgement. If these differ they discuss them and seek to persuade, but non-coercively (as the theory goes). Patient choice then requires the individual to be 'fully' informed. Thus, choice, perhaps, becomes both more rational and more valued. This is to give the doctor the role of enabling the patient to make choices. This requires new skills amongst both doctors and patients in a new era of medicine. We need to build the patient's ability to decide by enabling each to have the right to express themselves in terms of their values, to encourage self-esteem, to define good practice and to tie this to a system both of conflict-mediation and of sanction and redress. A flexible framework stated morally and facilitated practically, which will guide and empower both patients and health staff, too.

We need some care about language. Look back again to the geology of language. Consider the word 'compliance', with its encapsulation of 'will' and of patient yielding, with its paternalistic conception of the doctor–patient relationship in which an expert exercises autonomous power over a patient, defined (wrongly) as a non-expert. The ethics writer Soren Holm[43] has noted that to make progress we should abandon the conception of compliance. For if it is ultimately the patient who has to decide – on being duly informed and advised – then he cannot be non-compliant. The patient may be, as Holm says, non-collaborative, obstructive, foolish or stupid if he blatantly ignores decisions to which he is a leading party. But since these are the patient's own decisions and not the doctor's, this does not imply non-compliance.

The doctor and patient may, hopefully, share the same goal. But the issue of whether a doctor is responsible *to*, or responsible *for*, a patient prompts this fundamental enquiry about moral agency, individuality, self- and professional responsibility. This takes us into the encompassing, big-picture issues of what kind of a society we wish to construct, of how both improved health status and liberty are best rooted and of which dilemmas are necessarily irreconcilable.

There is a new element: the potency and cultural influence of new technology and multimedia, and of the World Wide Web. This promises to give patients access to information about what the practice is in other countries. This will continue to undermine the Bolam judgement, which itself depends on an idea which is rooted in a humanizing myth. That is, the notion that the doctor knows best, and that in a rational and consistent practice there is impersonally 'knowable' as the precondition for effective clinical medicine a best treatment for every disease and for every patient. This idea is simultaneously being challenged both by research and by the relativism of the patients' values in a world where there are few absolutes. There is the accumulating evidence, too, of the actuality of much diverse, unproved or ineffective diagnosis and therapy.

It seems essential to seek to reconcile all stakeholders around shared values and behaviours which are built on the idea that the patient does own the body and mind, has to manage with it, and in all cases of mental competence has to be in charge. Yet this is essential, I submit, to best enable modern health care to be delivered, because it will build self-esteem and meet the needs of morality. And, crucially, it will deliver a rapprochement of the values of medical professionals, and patients. This does, I agree, re-define the autonomy of the doctor so that it means someone who works within a value system which requires them to help patients find their own pathways.

Thus, doctor and nurse as geographers, as mappers of terrain, as delineators of ways to reach desirable goals, but not the ultimate determiners of those goals. Thus, the health professional's role is to help the individual to assert control over the factors which affect their lives, their health, their liberty. Thus, to become empowered rather than represented by an advocate, an agent or a proxy – unless they wish otherwise, which it should be their free decision to make. And so, to 'empowerment'.

The hammers of the piano: empowerment

Empowerment now bobs up in policy debate 'like eighteen hammers in a pianoforte', in Charles Dickens' vibrant phrase.

I have been discussing empowerment in the context of possession and dispossession, of control and its alternatives. My view is that the empowered user is vital for the development and transformation of modern health care and of modern mental health care – where there are many innovations, but where public concern about the balance between freedom and control exists. Rose Echlin[47] has shown recently how a release of imagination can equip professionals and mental health service users to develop together. It can be transformational. For people can select and will commit to and exercise choices that work for them, in terms of their values and beliefs. And if the patient is genuinely empowered the deficits in information, practice, audit, incentive and service which we see in the NHS will have to be recovered.

We need, I think, to agree that the issue about modern health care is not only that it is not primarily acute and elective hospital care. Nor is it primarily the care of the young, despite the bias of our society. Indeed it is going to become increasingly a health system preoccupied with the elderly (whose experience and wisdom we under-value and whose care we under-provide). As the Australian analysts Erica Bates and Helen Lapsley[48] noted, 'We are not organised to deal with groups of people whose illnesses are slow in onset and may never get better. Medical science has no effect on many of these conditions; it cures only very few; and it prolongs [life] ... the challenge is to set up support systems which will enable people to stay home rather than enter institutions'.

This is about chronic illnesses which are not necessarily life-threatening: arthritis, heart disease, high blood pressure, multiple sclerosis, diabetes, mental illness, dementia, stroke, disabling conditions which impede daily life which need continuing or recurrent care for many years. This is, of course, about helping people manage self-care and about helping people make life-style choices. This is crucial as the future pattern of health care becomes explicit. The future of health care is generally believed to be the significant burden of management of chronic illness in the community. Chiefly in the home – with only the very ill in hospital. Long-term care, which is getting longer term. Here, in particular, there are daunting challenges for the care of the mentally ill.

For this programme of care to succeed, the engaged self-aware, involved ('empowered') patient needs to be a cardinal objective of public policy. We must build self-esteem and shared management of treatments and of alternatives to treatment, including the individual deciding to do nothing in some circumstances, in accord with individual values which people can help make work by exercising their own choices. The fundamental and axiomatic point is that to such an agenda the informed, empowered patient is an essential partner in effective, appropriate, timely, safe and accessible health care whose *purposes* – as well as whose standards – they help to set, or which they set for themselves.

Myth and mystique: webs we make

A major difficulty is that not only are we all culturally bound, but many of our chains are iron-cast, within ourselves and by our own mind and hand.

The mystic role of medicine, the mystique of medical professionals, the humanizing myth of the certainty of solutions, the absence of self-belief in many patients – these are culture-bound concepts and psychic realities. So, too, is the restricted, indeed, the often willingly passive role of the patient and user of services. These historically bound concepts apparently reflect something fundamental in our evolved nature. Something, perhaps, rooted in our notions of the sacred and in our inevitable anxiety: we wish for the sacred and we feel its relevant anagram: we are scared. Max Weber said: 'Man is an animal suspended in webs of significance of his own making, in webs he has himself spun'.

Yet giving up our independence in the hope of security has produced dependence upon a system over which we feel we have no control. A system which in its diffuseness is unaccountable and often insensitive in fundamental details. We are not called upon – we do not call upon ourselves – as individuals to have power within ourselves. We need to take Stephen

Talbott's[49] advice (offered with regard to computers but key to health care systems): 'Our artifacts gain a life of their own, but it is, in a very real sense *our* life. We too easily ignore the ways in which we infuse these artifacts with the finespun web of our own, largely subconscious habits of thought. The need is to raise these habits to full consciousness, and then take responsibility for them'. The philologist Owen Barfield has noted that 'it is not man who made the myths, but the myths that made man'. Mystification and privilege are entwined; so, too, contrarily are mystery and the apparently willing lack of patient privilege. This is again to recognize that what matters is our 'inside', which is fundamental in our relations with the world 'outside'. I do not mean our physical inside, but our psychology, our expectations, our self-belief, our values, for want of a simpler word, our personal philosophy.

Any change, too, will rely on the psychological truth that the basis for any of us to know things is that they become transparent to us, that they become obvious to us. This obviousness has to be experienced from the 'inside' by an individual, so that the individual then begins to live within the self-supported (not system required) nature of their own thinking and action. We are embedded in our social structures, the more powerfully for resonating with our own unconscious. For we have a positive responsibility for what exists; it is not an accident.

Patient empowerment asks for a conscious relation to ourselves. For a wakefulness within ourselves. For the recognition that such an inner voice can alone prompt a responsible pursuit of better health care by the individual in their own terms. It is these internal, psychological propositions which are the basis for external changes. For responsibility comes from within. It cannot come from strategies handed down, though these might assist with some of the information which is needed to inform choice and change.

Responsibility cannot be 'delivered' or commanded. Responsibility is a cultural characteristic of an economic structure; it is not 'deliverable' either by paternalism or leadership. It derives instead from informed reflective duty and personal conduct which is self-directed. It is behaviour rooted in ownership, in private property rights, in individual rewards for good stewardship. That is, in the thought, knowledge and responsibility which is integral to living, which assists the process of learning, of education, of enabling the patient to experience themselves fully, to express personal values and expectations, to be equipped as an individual to make judgements.

Thus, to support self-esteem, to impact on health status, to build a better, more reflective, society, we need to free people to be better people, to carry personal responsibility and the moral values of society. This is not to call for isolated individualism – that is not the ideal. It is to call for individualism within a strengthened sense of solidarity in society. As David Green[50] has argued, this can only be attained by people voluntarily living under the same shared moral obligations, in self-awareness of what they want to do with their power. Indeed, devices for empowerment will only work if they give power to people to develop the capacity for self-possession and reflection within themselves. For morality and civilization can survive only in a society where individuals live in the true sense together – where they accept responsibility both for their own lives and for the lives of others closely tied to them, through bonds of common purpose and affection – as in families, friendships and small voluntary or jointly owned enterprises.

On this view, the lack of patient power is not merely correctable as a technical defect of a system. It is a fundamental problem about how we as individuals see ourselves and about who we choose to become. It co-exists, too, with the fact that ideals are often disguised interests.

A real revolution requires a process of education and preparation. This we should begin. For, if we do not do so, the existing mental regime will persist, and it will re-emerge as reforms 'settle down'. Berlin[3] cites Herzen's remark: 'One can't build a house for free people out of the bricks of a prison house'. As Berlin adds: 'to create a revolution before the people are ready, and before they know how to live in freedom, means that they will retain the old habits of the prisoners, and there will be no gain'.

This is, substantially, an issue about the status of particular kinds of knowledge.

It is, too, an endeavour which asks us to seek a form of relationship in which doctors are guided by a professional value system, with open accountability, but where the patient's autonomy and fundamental right to self-determination is acknowledged. This itself admits uncertainty, and may move us away from myth and mystique. For what doctors offer is not certain, but interpretative. Medicine is an interpretative science. Medicine gives advice, communicates judgements, offers an opinion on what is in the patient's best interests. This is not a counsel of absolute truth, even when some patients hope that it is.

And, as medicine offers the patient both interpretation and alternative courses of treatment, including the option of its refusal, we find we have underestimated the areas for choice and the capacity of patients to exercise choice. It is the patient, the recipient of advice, who has to take a decision if they so wish, for they have to be responsible for living with that choice in that mind and body. This is even more the case as we notice that medicine, indeed, may well involve the most intimate and invasive intrusion into someone else's body. They, patients, take the consequences.

If it is a fundamental moral requirement that agents must be responsible for themselves, it may be that it is doctors who should comply with the informed and considered wishes of their patients, and not the reverse. But doctors are their own moral agents, too. The helplessness and dependency of patients often encourages the idea that agents are justified in assuming responsibility for them. Yet, too, if long-term independence is an essential aim as we live longer we should challenge the necessity of coercive relationships, which damage liberty and which limit the potential of independent living. *En passant*, we could note the point, too, that patients with chronic disease can be as knowledgeable and as expert as the doctor who claims special knowledge and expertise. Certainly, too, for many conditions – diabetes, AIDS – the patient (or carer) soon becomes the foremost expert on his or her disease and on their experience of it and of its treatment.

There are other issues which I can only headline. For example, consumerism should not be thought to be a route to producing what one medical commentator, William Pickering,[51–53] has called the adoption by doctors of 'the role of helpless, tractable, even servile, instruments of their patients', for if they do consistent quality in medical practice will be beyond us. Equally, we should ask, how do doctors form their views of patients, how are doctors socialized, and what are the results? This urges us to pay attention to the structure within which students and residents learn. There is growing research on the effects and moral relevance (and limits to vision) of the human institution we know as medical training. We should ask, how do doctors form their views of patients, and what are the results?

Training creates highly structured anticipations about practice and patients, about the professional's sense of self, and about what Langdon Winner[9] calls 'associated language games that are part of human culture'. It is a recognized and special problem of medical training – and subsequently of the individual's experience of the services received – that the patient becomes harder to see as a person, in a morally effective way as training progresses. Indeed, there is an intrinsic tension between the necessary objectivity of medical training and attending to the patient's subjectivity. It is vital, however, that what doctors do to doctors in socialization and training should not be done to patients. And that the socialization of doctors, and career progression, is changed diametrically by a new focus on consumer priority. Patients should refuse the impersonality and insist on a humanized medicine. It will be difficult for doctors to respond.

As one commentator, Judith Andre,[54] says: 'Institutions shape perception; they make some things visible, they mark things as important; they show what is possible'. As Andre writes: 'Training years do not exist in isolation: they are meant to prepare people for a profession practised in a certain way'. Yet we want doctors to develop an understanding of patients as persons – 'complexly biological but always more than that; not always co-operative, not always fixable, but always the centre of their own lives'. We want to legitimize patients as choosers, with sanctions. We need to change training.

Subjectivity and quality of life questions (which patients alone can determine for themselves) need to be given a new primacy. As Good and Good[55] noted, during medical training students reconstruct their view of the world so that patients become bodies, with little stress on their social and personal characteristics. The interior of the individual, their thoughts, experiences, personality recede from view, for the interior in the lab. is tissue, cells, organs. Doctors need our help in re-realizing the humanistic values which, we hope, motivated them to go to medical school.

Too often, too, the emphasis on the concept of empowerment remains that of 'involving' the public in planning. The emphasis on 'training' the public also offers the hazard that the public continues to be seen from a managerial perspective.

It is clear that Alan Langlands, the NHS Chief Executive, is committed to the idea of patient partnership and to real change in how the NHS relates to its users. But I retain anxieties about this project, even if it is seen as much more than an 'initiative'. I still wish to ask whether patient partnership will create the taste for patient empowerment, will it create the taste by which it is to be enjoyed, will the consumer be empowered to insist? Will 'partnership' genuinely open up the system to a new psychological character, and to new conceptions of meaning? Certainly, the policy does not satisfy the precondition for which I argue, that the consumer must *prevail* and that professionals be seen as service-providers in a partnership which they do not control. In developing a new public culture, and new ways to relate to our public institutions, we need to be very alert to official documents which (in the words of a critic of literature) may seem to ordinary patients (if conceived as consumers who must prevail over producers) 'so intensely written, so little seen, known or felt'.[56]

The psychological reality of health care is that even in a more open 'partnership', the patient necessarily bears all of the risk. All staff actions, all organizational values, all psychological assumptions, all definitions of actions, must respond to this insight. It is a key question whether or not partnership as a concept can help us imagine a new world, and then to engage with it in the most profound ways in terms of who we conceive 'patients' and professionals to be. James Joyce tells us in *Ulysses* that these arguments are about 'those big words ... which make us so unhappy'.[57] That is, belief and faith, power and control, freedom, choice and responsibility. Yet we need to be open about what are necessary tensions and not submerge these in 'partnership'. That is, if we are to move forward outside a received blanket of blandness and apparent ease. Adaptations will be very difficult to accomplish and very disturbing to manage. But if we do not openly recognize the cause of tensions and face up to them we will have no understanding of how to manage the divergence between theoretical and actual results.

We are necessarily dealing with painful states of mind and of being, focused on power and control. The issue of the genuinely empowered (and financially resourced) service-user is the central concern of the day for public institutions. It is, too, the axis of fulfilment for change, in this troubling territory. These are fundamental challenges to the creative imagination. It is not sufficient to pull out new leaves at the end of an established and familiar dining table, in the terms of Twemlow in *Our Mutual Friend*.[56] For we need an entirely new 'article' (to use a Dickensian word). Ultimately, patients themselves must be able to decide how much power they have and on which terms they wish (if at all) to be partners.

Empowerment, and the punctuation mark

A humble item of English punctuation is important in this cultural analysis. This is the punctuation mark. Words and concepts in initial quotes, such as 'wrong', 'choice', 'expert', 'knowledge', and 'certainty' and, most essentially, 'empowerment' and its Antipodean opposite, 'partnership', which seems at first hearing to be the echo but is not the image of autonomy.

The list of words and concepts in quotation marks is a list with an ecology. For these words embody confining cultural expectations. They name not 'facts' but intentions. They predictively label in the actual act of inventing spaces and possibilities. They give cultural circulation to specific strategies about modes of knowing and being. Notably, about who has which power and knowledge to exercise in which space, with which valid mental attitudes and in which direction of travel. These words set the limits of patient significance, of sanction, and of self-reflection. For the individual, they limit oneself in experiencing oneself. They are an assertion about possession. They limit what the NHS can hope to achieve. Revisionist changes in words are essential to permit and to articulate changes in knowledge and action, to release and achieve new punctuations.

We can see that patient empowerment is a big-sky issue. It prompts many to run for cover, since it opens up everything that has not yet been tackled by reform: personally defined quality, standards, social consent, professional accountability, contract, selection, education, socialization, incentive, reward.

A word here about words. About what they conceal and reveal. For language consists of fossilized metaphors. We are working with ideas which are conceptualized with words. Words locate and conceptualize places, attitudes, expectations. They encompass totemic meanings. Significantly, language can offer a process of subversion of the momentum of events. As E Annie Proulx[58] warns, we must be careful, too, of 'mistaking the fact for the idea'. In 1995 the NHS Executive began with a search for an 'empowerment' strategy. This has now been converted into the less salient, because less threatening, 'partnership' project. But under either flag, in a flurry of study and discussion, there remains the risk that 'patient empowerment' could become what the anthropologist Clifford Geertz[26] called 'a protocol sentence', apparently descriptive of a concept in use, but not an action that works.

We need to see this if we are to re-define cultural frameworks to empower doctors and patients with common values. 'Partnership' apparently associates the individual patient with power. Yet it does not add to patient autonomy, with its capacity for comparison – Hume's definition of reason. It deducts from it. It does so by enmeshing it in a net of associations which rely on superior (rather than just different) professional experience. This is stated as medical knowledge (rather than as a mix of technique and values) which lives in effective command and veto over both resources, politics and definitions of what determines health status.

There is little hint that the patient should be enabled to feel dominance over the situation. The key, instead, I suggest, is to equip the individual with sanctions and control over budgetary allocation as an incentive to effective clinical practice. For the key for the individual is direct *personal* leverage over which clinician, which treatment, where – over specific service delivery decisions. We need *specific devices which are intended to empower patients as the principal objective of public policy for effective health care – delivering the objective that empowerment is the outcome*. Real, practical devices for the 'empowerment' of 'choice', which could both deliver it and measure what happens.

We do, I think, have to agree that health care is an example of market failure. That is, if we do not regulate the market then supply creates its own demand, in a situation of differential consumer and producer knowledge. Thus, the role of the doctor historically as the agent of the patient and adviser on consumption. Thus, the role of government in moderating demand, controlling over-supply and controlling increases in costs.

However, within this understanding, my principal institutional innovation is patient fundholding (PFH), with the patient as purchaser, advised by the GP. Again, this returns us to self-transformation, self-understanding and choice. The challenge is to develop this whilst avoiding the problems of moral hazard, client and treatment exclusion of the Health Maintenance Organization and of unnecessary service and higher costs of a fee-for-service system. If we genuinely do want empowerment and consumer choice, there is no alternative but for patients to be given the compelling power of money. This will wrest substantial control over financial mechanisms away from managers as well as from physicians. This need not, of course, breach politically determined budgetary ceilings – or global budgets – at regional or national levels. But it is likely to supplement those budgets personally.

'Partnership', even 'empowerment', as yet, suggest nothing of this. As a technique it has, instead, been viewed by the NHS as a technique of legitimacy, not of discovery. The NHS Executive discussion has been an avoidance and a substitution. This is inevitable in a political marketplace. The concepts and the language employed make assumptions which are fundamentally disempowering. The approach taken and the language are signs of avoidance and of the inability of those inside a system to scrutinize it in the language of those outside the system. It is not enough to introduce partnerships. The consumer must *prevail* over the producer, which will require individual payment. In my proposal this will be derived from tax-based finance which is already allocated by the health authorities via their 'agent', the GP.

There are ten characteristics of a template which would show that patients are empowered.

1　That they control budgetary allocation.
2　That there is price-conscious quality choice.
3　That patients are expected to predominate in decision-making.
4　That patients control the agenda.
5　That there are no barriers to information.
6　That 'information' becomes knowledge, for leverage.
7　That the NHS helps people ask the *hard* questions, which will make up *its* deficits.
8　That narrative experience is shared easily between service users *before* they accept treatment.
9　That patients' own expectations of their roles change, as they assume it is reasonable to ask for what they want instead of being preoccupied with guilt.
10　That patients themselves decide how much power they are to have, instead of professionals and managers deciding how much power to grant them.

All ten are essential if empowerment is to be real and meaningful. There needs especially to be good information on the patient's condition, good information in public on what does what well and access to the narrative experience of other patients 'like me'. Devices for individual leverage are then the rubric of empowerment as people deal with the consequences of choice instead of handing over power.

It is ideas which pose issues; it is ideas which produce critical contrast; it is ideas which spark the individual to make life choices. But it is *devices* which deliver the change. And so, like the pursuing Sheriff with the white boater, hunting Butch Cassidy and the Sundance Kid, we must keep a relentless focus on empowering devices. Notably, specific data and money, with decisions informed by self-realization and supported by the social determination that this enables a better (and, indeed kinder) society.

We need, too, to encourage and support one another to hold on to what Dickens called 'the natural feelings of the heart', our individuality, our emotions and feelings, our sensitivities, values and beliefs in every situation in which we find ourselves. In each health care location, we need to express our questions in these terms and to make up our own answers if at all possible as we make up our own minds. We need to hold on to our sense of self (which is not the same as a sense of selfishness), as we pose questions and make choices. Otherwise, the health care system will continue to define health and our individuality will merely be absorbed into the system which does not value the particular. For the risk of each institutional situation is, as Dickens voices in *Bleak House*, 'we are made parties to it, and *must* be parties to it, whether we like it or not'. Instead, professionals must let go of their grip on the processes.

We do, of course, need the epic comforts. But we also need the intimate. The intimate, personal picture is the requirement to ensure that all receive effective care *which they help to define in advance* as we empower all as individuals in terms of their own values, beliefs and choices. We need this both in those situations which pose excruciating dilemmas which we have been considering and in 'ordinary' acute and mental and community care where 'empowerment' can much enhance life. We need to remind ourselves, too, of what Ronald Dworkin said: 'We live our whole lives in the shadow of death ... it is also true that we die in the shadow of our whole lives'.

'If I am not for me ...'

I draw the last rap on my drum from a lecture by the Harvard geologist and evolutionist Stephen Jay Gould,[59] with which he accepted the Edinburgh Gold Medal in 1990.

In this piece, *The Individual in Darwin's World*, Gould suggests many interconnections which are our concern as we consider who owns our bodies, as we reconsider the relevance and reach of health policy, as we seek to cohere common values for uncommon health gains. For he deals with the concept of individuality. He queries our assumptions about the nature of the world. He notices our hopes about the world and the contrast with the observed nature of Nature. He discusses the centrality of personhood and our hopes for reassurance in the world we know. He talks of the plain-language implications of frightening facts – including the idea that science is not necessarily an inexorable march to truth through the collection of objective information. He focuses on contingency and admits uncertainties.

Gould says: 'We aggregate into collectivities. But each of us is different from everyone else and undoubtedly a personality unto himself'. And: 'the growing ties among us, that universal brotherhood and sisterhood to which we aspire, is perfectly good biology, and the enlarged notion of individuality is not just outdated liberal hope or mushy romanticism. Of course, I hope we never abrogate our focus on bodies as well, if only for that ultimate of political reasons, namely that we weep for the inhumanity of some systems that did not cherish the worth of individual bodies, but did flourish for a time nonetheless. Still, I would repeat in conclusion that it is not outdated liberalism or mushy romanticism but perfectly good biology to say, in that most famous statement from [the Jewish] tradition, as Rabbi Hillel has said: 'If I am not for myself, then who shall be for me? But if I am for myself alone, then what am I?'

References

1   Erikson E (1958) The nature of clinical evidence. In: *Evidence and inference.* (ed. D Learner). The Free Press of Glencoe, Illinois.

2   Bradbury M (1993) *Introduction to* Nathaniel Hawthorne: *The Blithedale Romance.* Everyman Edition. JM Dent, London.

3   Berlin I (1969) *Four essays on liberty.* OUP, Oxford.

4   Hayek F (1960) *The constitution of liberty.* University of Chicago Press, Chicago.

5   Mill JS (1991) On Liberty. In: *On liberty and other essays.* (ed. J Gray). OUP, Oxford.

6   Jahanbegloo R (1992) *Conversations with Isaiah Berlin: recollections of an historian of ideas.* Peter Halbon, London.

7   Goffman E (1959) *The presentation of self in everyday life.* Doubleday, New York.

8   Singer P (1995) *Rethinking life and death: the collapse of our traditional ethics.* OUP, Oxford.

9   Winner L (1986) *The whale and the reactor: a search for limits in an age of high technology.* Chicago University Press, Chicago.

10 Annan N (1982) *Isaiah Berlin: personal impressions.* OUP, Oxford.

11 Gray J (1995) *Berlin.* Modern Masters Series. Fontana Press, London.

12   Flaubert G (translated by G Wall) (1994) *The dictionary of received ideas*. Penguin, London.

13   Raz J (1994) *Ethics in the public domain*. Clarendon Press, Oxford.

14   *Airedale NHS Trust v. Bland CA*. House of Lords. 19 February 1993, 2 WLR 350.

15   Daley J (1996) Where's mercy in such killings? In: *The Daily Telegraph*, 16 April 1996.

16   Clough S (1996) NHS seeks to let man 'die with dignity'. In: *The Daily Telegraph*, 18 April 1996.

17   Dyer C (1996) Judge grants end to 'living death'. In: *The Guardian*, 4 April 1996.

18   Dyer C (1996) Judge will rule on treatment. In: *The Guardian*, 18 April 1996.

19   Lightfoot E (1996) Judge will rule on right to life. In: *The Sunday Times*, 14 April 1996.

20   Bunyan N (1996) Son admits giving drug overdose to mother in agony with cancer. In: *The Daily Telegraph*, 13 April 1996.

21   Frost B (1996) Son explains why he ended pain. In: *The Times*, 13 April 1996.

22   Anon (1996) Parents win right to let baby die. In: *Yorkshire Post*, 4 April 1996.

23   Berlin I (1991) *The crooked timber of humanity*. Fontana Press, London.

24   Keane J (1995) *Tom Paine: a political life*. Bloomsbury, London.

25   Belton N (1996) Candied porkers: British scorn of the scientific. In: *Cultural babbage: technology, time and invention* (eds F Spufford and J Uglow). Faber and Faber, London.

26   Geertz C (1993) *The interpretation of cultures: selected essays*. (2nd ed.). Fontana Press, London.

27   Buchanan J (1975) *The limits of liberty: between anarchy and leviathon*. University of Chicago Press, Chicago.

28   Buchanan J and Tullock G (1965) *The calculus of consent*. University of Michigan Press, Ann Arbor.

29   Buchanan J (ed.) (1978) *The economics of politics*. Institute of Economic Affairs, London.

30   Shears R (1996) The world's first case of legal euthanasia. In: *The Daily Mail*, 18 April 1996.

31 Alcorn G (1996) Why she wants to die by computer. In: *The Daily Telegraph*, 19 April 1996.

32 Evans RG (1990) The dog in the night-time: medical practice variations and health policy. In: *The challenges of medical practice variations* (eds TV Anderson and G Mooney). Economic Issues in Health Care Series. Macmillan Press, London.

33 McKeown T (1979) *The role of medicine: dream, mirage or nemesis?* Basil Blackwell, Oxford.

34 McKinley JB and McKinley SM (1977) The questionable contribution of medical measures to the decline of mortality in the United States in the Twentieth Century. *Milbank Memorial Fund Quarterly, Health and Society.* **55**(3).

35 Sagan LA (1987) *The health of nations.* Basic Books, New York.

36 Tenner E (1996) *Why things bite back: technology and the revenge effect.* Alfred A Knopf, New York.

37 Evans RG, Barer ML and Marmot R (1994) *Why are some people healthy and others not?* Aldine de Gruyter, New York.

38 Faulkner W (1951) *Requiem for a nun.* Penguin, Harmondsworth.

39 Hersey J (1987) *Blues.* Random House, New York.

40 Carter P (1987) *The road to Botany Bay: an exploration of landscape and history.* Alfred A Knopf, New York.

41 Kant I (translated by NK Smith) (1929) *Critique of pure reason.* Macmillan, London.

42 Loewy EH (1991) Involving patients in do not resuscitate (DNR) decisions: an old issue raising its ugly head. *J. Med. Ethics* **17**(3): 156–80.

43 Holm S (1993) What is wrong with compliance? *J. Med. Ethics* **19**(2): 108–10.

44 Fairbairn G (1991) Enforced death: enforced life. *J. Med. Ethics* **17**(3): 144–9.

45 *Bolam v. Friern Hospital Management Committee.* 1957, 1 WLR 582 (Queen's Bench Division).

46 Savelescu J (1995) Rational non-interventional paternalism: why doctors ought to make judgements of what is best for their patients. *J. Med. Ethics* **21**(6): 327–31.

47 Echlin R with Buck J (1995) *Partners in change: care planning in mental health services.* The King's Fund Centre, London.

48   Bates E and Lapsley H (1985) *The health machine: the impact of medical technology*. Penguin, Victoria, Australia.

49   Talbott SL (1995) *The future does not compute: transcending the machines in our midst*. O'Reilly & Associates, Sebastopol, California.

50   Green DG (1996) *Community without politics: a market approach to welfare reform*. Institute of Economic Affairs, Health and Welfare Unit, London.

51   Pickering W (1996) Does medical treatment mean patient benefit? *Lancet* **347**: 379–80.

52   Pickering W (1993) Patient satisfaction: an imperfect measurement of quality medicine. *J. Med. Ethics* **19**: 121–2.

53   Pickering W (1991) A nation of people called patients. *J. Med. Ethics* **17**: 91–2.

54   Andre J (1992) Learning to see: moral growth during medical training. *J. Med. Ethics* **18**: 148–52.

55   Good M and Good BJ (1989) Disabling practitioners: hazards of learning to be a doctor in American medical education. *Am. J. Orthopsychiatry* **59**(2): 303–9.

56   Gill S (ed.) (1985) *Our mutual friend* by Charles Dickens. Classics edition. Penguin, London, p. 12.

57   Joyce J (1992) *Ulysses*. Penguin, Harmondsworth, p. 38.

58   Proulx EA (1993) *The shipping news*. Fourth Estate, London.

59   Gould SJ (1990) *The individual in Darwin's world: the second Edinburgh Medal Address*. Weidenfeld & Nicholson, London.

Other sources

Anon (1996) *Advance statements about future medical treatment: a guide for patients*. The Patients Association, London.

Anon (1996) Coma woman allowed to die. In: *The Guardian*, 23 April 1996.

Anon (1996) It's your body ... In: *Health Which?*, April 1996.

Anon (1994) *Living wills: guidance for nurses*. Issues in nursing and health leaflet series no. 4. Royal College of Nursing, London.

Bentall RP (1992) A proposal to classify happiness as a psychiatric disorder. *J. Med. Ethics* **18**(2): 93–102.

British Medical Association (1993) *Guidelines on the treatment of patients in a persistent vegetative state*. BMA, London.

Brodie I (1996) US courts uphold right to assisted suicide. In: *The Times*, 9 April 1996.

Campbell AG and McHaffie HE (1995) Prolonging life and allowing death: infants. *J. Med. Ethics* 21(6): 339–44.

Clark B (1979) *Whose life is it anyway?* Dodd Mead, New York.

Collis JS (1978) *Living with a stranger: a discourse on the human body.* Macdonald and Janes, London.

Collis JS (1975) *The worm forgives the plough.* Penguin, London.

Cornwell J (1996) Back from the dead. In: *The Sunday Times Magazine*, 2 June 1996. (*Discusses the experiences of carers and patients with a special focus on the Royal Hospital for Neurodisability in Putney, London.*)

Devlin P (1965) *The enforcement of morals.* OUP, Oxford.

European Commission (1995) *The European Union and biomedical and health research.* IOS Press, Amsterdam. (On the BIOMED 1 Programme.)

Giacino GT and Zasler ND (1995) Outcome following severe brain injury: the comatose, vegetative and minimally responsive patient. *J. Head Trauma Rehabil.* 10: 20–56.

Gormally L (1993) Definition of personhood: implications for the care of PVS patients. *Ethics and Medicine*, 9.3.93.

Gormally L (1993) *Euthanasia, clinical practice and the law.* Submission to the Select Committee of the House of Lords on Medical Ethics.

Grubb A, Walsh P, Lambe N *et al.* (1996) Survey of British clinicians' views on management of patients in persistent vegetative state. *Lancet* 348: 35–40.

Hall C (1996) Disagree with voluntary euthanasia ... but don't deny the right to me. In: *The Daily Telegraph*, 27 September 1996.

Hughes J (1995) Ultimate justification: Wittgenstein and medical ethics. *J. Med. Ethics* 21(1): 25–30.

Jennett B and Plum F (1972) Persistent vegetative state after brain damage: a syndrome in search of a name. *Lancet* i: 734–47.

Kirby M (1995) Patients' rights: why the Australian courts have rejected 'Bolam'. *J. Med. Ethics* 21(1): 5–8.

Mabbott JD (1967) *The state and the citizen.* (2nd ed.) Hutchinson, London.

Martin GL (1996) Right to die Act gives choice of drugs. In: *The Daily Telegraph*, 25 May 1996.

McMillan RC (1995) Responsibility *to* or *for* in the physician-patient relationship? *J. Med. Ethics* 21(2): 112–15.

Multi-Society Task Force Report on PVS (1994) Medical aspects of the persistent vegetative state. *N. Engl. J. Med.* **330**: 1499–1508, 1572–9.

NHS Executive (1996) *Patient partnership: building a collaborative partnership*. Department of Health, Leeds.

NHS Executive (1995) *Priorities and planning guidance for the NHS: 1996/97*. Department of Health, Leeds.

New York State Task Force on Life and The Law (1994) *When death is sought: assisted suicide and euthanasia in the medical context*. NYSTFLL, New York.

Norden M (1995) Whose life is it anyway? A study in respect of autonomy. *J. Med. Ethics* **21**(3): 179–83.

Phillips M and Dawson J (1985) *Doctors' dilemmas: medical ethics and contemporary science*. The Harvester Press, Brighton.

Report of the Select Committee on Medical Ethics of the House of Lords, 31 January 1994.

Royal College of General Practitioners (1996) The permanent vegetative state. *J. R. Coll. Phys.* **30**: 119–21.

Roszak T (1994) *The cult of information: a neo-Luddite treatise on high-tech, artificial intelligence and the art of true thinking*. (2nd ed.) University of California Press, Berkeley.

Seldon A (1990) *Capitalism*. Blackwell, Oxford.

Senate of Canada (1995) *Of life and death*. Report of the Special Senate Committee on Euthanasia and Assisted Suicide.

Simons M (1996) Australia's day of deliverance. In: *The Guardian*, 18 May 1996.

Spiers J (1996) I have a wish, an anxiety and an analysis (revitalizing the role of the patient). *Health Care Today* **39**: 38–42.

Spiers J (1996) But will it work *for me*, doctor? In: *But will it work, doctor?* King's Fund, London/NHS Executive.

Spiers J (1996) 'Only a novel!' Jane Austen, hypertext and the story of patient power. In: *Sense and sensibility in health care* (ed. M Marinker). BMJ Publishing, London.

Spiers J (1995) *The invisible hospital and the secret garden: an insider's commentary on the NHS reforms*. Radcliffe Medical Press, Oxford.

Spiers J *'The prison of awe': patients and power*. In preparation.

White C (1996) Let coma woman wife die in peace, rules judge. In: *The Daily Telegraph*, 25 April 1996.

Afterword

We have had five years of health reform in Britain. And, as Berlin says, 'The oak cannot return to the condition of the acorn'.[1] We need now to go on to empowerment and to a new ethical structure which can accommodate the new medicine. This entails a moral framework which can bear the weight of change and command the assent of society. This is a difficult request. We would each like all's well to end well, so that, as Shakespeare says in the eponymous play, 'health shall live free, and sickness freely die'.[2] But how is this to be achieved?

I have argued that empowerment is at the root of necessary change, since its branches encompass self-esteem, self-responsibility and self-realization. Further, as we are told in *Bleak House*, 'Our plain course, however, under good report and evil report, and all kinds of prejudice ... is to have everything openly carried out'.[3]

There *is* a crisis concerning patient empowerment. The requirement remains the successful introduction of a basic alphabet of change: A, for attitude; B, for behaviour; C, for capacity to change. Behaviour, which breeds behaviour, has to change if attitudes are to alter since experience creates belief. These are especially significant problems of moral growth and socialization in medical training, the terms of which must change in response to patient empowerment, as Judith Andre's important study in part elucidates (and which other recent studies disappointingly overlook or under-estimate).[4] It is not clear how this can be achieved by politicians, nor by civil servants or health care managers.[5] There would seem to be a special role that only patients and service users can play. This realization proceeds in parallel with other changes, notably the apparent recession of faith in conventional lobbying and politics. Our supply-side changes, too, have isolated the 'proxy' agent, whose legitimacy is open to question. We need to consider carefully where the legitimate voice is to be heard, about how to see, what to do and why. Where is the authentic report to be found on what is going on, and with which results? Where is the authorized development, approved locally and properly accounted?

I have questioned the new NHS 'partnership strategy'. Certainly it is possible to argue that this is a beginning and that direct and valuable results may be generated. These may be a direct result of a process which has begun, rather than of specific policies. However, we still know little about the value that proxies add. Nor is it at all obvious how doctors share the two most vital elements – knowledge and risk. These are integral to any partnership. We have a problem about what we mean by 'knowledge'. And the concept of 'risk' is problematic. For 'risk' is something which it is just not possible for anyone to share with the patient, who receives the treatment, owns the body and has to live with (or die with) the results. Theodore Roszak reminds us, too, to be alert to how words (in my terms, such as 'partnership' or 'empowerment') are used. He says: 'Words that come to mean everything may finally mean nothing; yet their very emptiness may allow them to be filled with a mezmerizing glamour'.[6] We notice, too, that patients still report that they are spoken to with patronage, condescension or childishness, as Dickens says, 'like little spelling books'.[7]

There remains, too, the issue of 'demand management'. It may be that in a service innocent of cost-conscious choice this is inconsolably unmanageable. Expectations will rise, despite policies which call for 'sssh!'. However, the concepts of control direct our eyes to the wrong peaks. For it may instead be that the informed, self-reflective, self-responsible service user (who is asked to make evaluated choices between options, whose objectives they help establish) will be a less demanding user of services. And, often, thus a healthier person. This bears more consideration than the strategy of 'partnership' seems to offer and reflect. This is to argue, too, that health care must move from its politically-derived, almost obsessional emphasis on volume, to more openly enquire about those triggers of self-esteem which themselves locate good health.

There is a crisis, too, in ethics. For moral decision-making turns on the axis of autonomy and self-realization. This has coincided with new medical opportunities and with the re-assertion of individuality and choice. These are technical, social and psychological changes which have impelled new social, ethical and legal attitudes. For example, the sanctity of life ethic was first and directly challenged by an appeal to quality of life arguments in debates about abortion. These changes in ethical thinking are a response, too, to a decline in religious authority. And, to a fuller (if uncomfortable) understanding of the animal nature and inheritance of our species. Together, these are formidable challenges to our evolutionary history by contrast with our 'divine nature' and the notion of God as the great architect of our being.

Stephen Jay Gould, for example, has shown how the pageant of evolution has been a series of staggeringly improbable events which are unlikely to recur could the historical tape be re-run.[8] And, changes in ethical views have acknowledged the realizations implied by quantum physics. This sees an expansively bizarre cosmology, a Universe of nemesis, a vast expanding emptiness in which the address 'Earth' is at best suburban. For we are located in a rather minor Milky Way, despite its temporary blaze of the light of a hundred billion stars.

Peter Singer is notable in his subtle but purposeful discussions of how we confront a fundamental and unavoidable crisis in morality and ethics. Singer identifies the context of this crisis as the decline in the explanatory and persuasive power of the traditional western ethic. This stated the intrinsic sanctity and worth of all human life *irrespective* of its quality. Singer guides our understanding of the necessary Copernican shift to an ethics openly emphasizing the quality of life. This displacement is essential and not merely expedient, but it is only being raggedly achieved. However, he argues, it is as important as the supplantation of Ptolemy.

A more traditional ethics emphasizes our centrality. Meanwhile, the Universe cools towards its dismal conclusion of a probable heat-death as resources tend to finite and time tends to infinity. Or order gives way to entropy. And physicists enhance discontinuity with the intuitively odd notion that before the big bang there was *no* before. That the big bang was the ultimate beginning of all physical things: space, time, matter, and energy. That where there is no time there can be no causation in the ordinary sense. Thus, we are no longer the clear reason for it all. Our individuality marks little time in time itself. Or, coming down to earth itself, we have Singer's own note of the clash of science and the Judaeo-Christian culture: 'If we are the reason why everything else was made, why do we have such an undistinguished address?'

The moral and ethical challenge is to retain our grounds for emphasizing the sanctity of life, even without the confident centrality of people in a divinely designed Universe. We have seen already that, like the Universe of infinite and entropic emptiness, our personal beginning and our end are deeply intertwined. For many of us the ethical question includes how should we express our lives by influencing our final three minutes. Daily we struggle with ethical, legal and practical anomalies. We have not yet constructed a satisfactory alternative ethic by which we can be guided beyond the fragmentation of our moral inheritance. In England, the tragic Anthony Bland case most notably dramatized these dilemmas, as did the case of Nancy Cruzan in the USA.[9] This was essentially a debate about what it is to be a human being. The judgement in that case effectively said that although the organs of the body were alive (excepting the cortex) the 'person' in that case was effectively dead. The critical capacity here was determined to be that of being able to feel, to process information, to experience. Continuing debates about voluntary and involuntary euthanasia, about the status of the fetus, about advance directives, about what we mean by life and by death pose the same questions.

In Britain, we now regularly confront new and sensitive ethical cases in the courts. These concern individual actions in the most sensitive of personal (and thus of societal) situations. In one week in October 1996, for example, we saw the case of a bed-ridden brother suffering from the incurable degenerative Huntington's Disease, who asked his brother to suffocate him.[10] Second, there was the case of a young widow (Mrs Diane Blood) seeking to have her dead husband's frozen sperm implanted to try for a baby, but denied because written consent was absent. The husband had died suddenly of meningitis. Whilst he was unconscious sperm had been taken from the husband and stored by the Infertility Research Trust pending the resolution of the legal issues. Mrs Blood applied for a judicial review, in order to produce the child the couple had been seeking prior to his illness. Where did the rights of autonomy and of regulation lie?[11] Intensive care units and the Family Division of the High Court especially are becoming exposed and sensitized arenas for the resolution of anguishing, bewildering and often tragic and contradictory hopes.

Euthanasia is an ever-present challenge. The choices now being made by some Australian, Dutch and Oregon citizens are asked for by many of our own citizens. These possible options cause concern and anxiety amongst others, who question the confidence that the elderly will place in medicine and that they may feel they will have a 'duty to die'. Advocates of voluntary euthanasia say that to continue to live in further predictable and irresolvable suffering in life is insufficient compensation when set against the oblivion of death. Many clearly fear intolerable suffering more than death; they prefer an escape from pain into nothingness, into a 'state' in which there is no 'next'. In these circumstances, as Bacon noted, 'therefore death is no terrible enemy'. The autonomous wish here is often for control and an integral reflection of self-realization as it has been lived in life itself, of which death is a part. We are not yet reconciled as a society to such an ethic, despite Christian convictions and those influenced by Hindu and Buddhist belief in a cycle of birth and death. Yet it is these most serious dilemmas of practice which we need to sort out in a new ethics and a new morality – pressingly, as very many more of us live on to endure Alzheimer's and other degenerative diseases. We need to sustain social consent, discipline practice and bear the weight of innovation.

It seems to me that the guidance we have from Dworkin and from Singer is taking us on the appropriate track. As ethics shift, the law needs to codify new opportunities and to regulate defensible positions. One large part of our emphasis should be on the proper goals of medicine. That is, those of treating treatable disease with a fundamental concern for compassionate and responsive choice, including the ending of treatment and perhaps the non-criminal ending of life if that is what the individual wishes. For kindness and the opportunity to reduce intolerable pain and suffering are fundamental to respect for the intrinsic sanctity of life and for the personal values

of how to live and die.[12] Good law should be nimble an
realization, the avoidance of state coercion and proper reg
the vulnerable. The law should respond to the emphasis gi\
reverence for the intrinsic value and dignity of all human
in terms of its nature and quality and in terms of the sel_~   _{~, ~. ~ne}
individual.

It seems that many, including senior Law Lords in their recent decision-making, now take a relativistic position which asks what the life being so valued is actually like. This shift poses many risks. It asks us to seek to re-shape our ethics to enable lives to be lived in the fullest humanity and in honourable mutual understanding, but some of these lines for action remain difficult to draw. Close regulation, and the protection of the vulnerable, is essential. So, too, as Dr William Pickering has pointed out, is the necessity of responsibility: for people need to think about these problems for themselves and not just to give them away to doctors to deal with on their behalf.[13]

We are increasingly asking about fundamentals which are more elusive than we expect them to be. What do we mean by death and how do we know it has occurred? When does a human being die? When should medicine stop trying to prevent this? How is the moral community to be protected and who are its members? Does membership arise at conception and when is that? Or at birth, or only if the child has certain agreed and given characteristics? The law must define. It must, too, regulate change, practice, motive and manner of action. We need a much more satisfactory legal and ethical framework for soundly based choices concerning what it means to bring into being, prolong or end life. We need to sort out when, how, and on what grounds a human life has a claim to protection, and from whom (including ourselves?).

My argument is for an ethical and moral code of compassion and choice, of autonomy and realism to support self-realization. And for open-eyed honesty as we consider the laws concerning voluntary and involuntary euthanasia, abortion, the treatment of anencephalic and cortically-dead infants, the treatment of patients in a persistent vegetative state and those who are comatose but whose cortex still receives blood. The issue is partly that of who is to be included in the moral community, who is to be accorded moral status and protection, who excluded, on what grounds, and to what purpose? We must re-examine these fundamentals about choice and autonomy (including the problem of whether autonomy and best-interests coincide), of who owns our bodies and who should make decisions about our life and death. How we conduct this debate, and how we release the transforming powers of self-realization and choice, of course impacts more widely on the overall nature of society. There is always a big sky.

efinitions

To begin with, we need clear and unambiguous new definitions of when human life begins and ends. Existing definitions do not serve.

For example, brain death is accepted as death for all legal purposes, but it is not sufficient to guide satisfactory practice. The Tony Bland case (whose body was warm and breathing but whose higher brain had turned to fluid), together with the similar and earlier Nancy Cruzan case in the USA, asked us to consider this issue.[14] For neither Tony Bland nor Nancy Cruzan had the capacity any longer to ever recover consciousness. More precise medical knowledge unmistakeably demonstrated that since damage to the higher brain (the cerebral cortex, responsible for consciousness) was irreversible, there would be no 'waking up'. Yet since the brain stem and central nervous system was functioning, both patients were freely breathing whilst artificially fed. They were in a 'persistent vegetative state'. Their families wished this to be lawfully stopped.

In Britain this request was eventually granted by the House of Lords sitting judicially. It was denied by the US Supreme Court in the case of Nancy Cruzan, in the absence of convincing evidence that Cruzan's wishes were known or knowable. In America, judges emphasized personal autonomy. In Britain the judges decided differently and emphasized quality of life. Each asked what was in the best interest of the patient.

The new term, brain-dead, has emerged in response to technology. For modern procedures have made possible the impossible. They have enabled a dead human being with a disabled and non-functioning brain, whose heart nevertheless still beats, to continue to 'exist'. Blood circulation and oxygenation of the 'dead' body is maintained by technology. This was the situation of both Tony Bland and Nancy Cruzan. Neither could meaningfully be said to be a burden on themselves. Neither, however, had any medical prospect of becoming themselves again. In these cases, the intelligent, sensate, experiential adult had disappeared. In these cases the essential human individual and their life had disappeared. There remained what Christopher Pallis has called 'a heart-beating cadaver'.[15] Their tragedy lay in the arbitrary and senseless loss of all the possibilities of life and yet without the dignity of death. Tony Bland 'survived' as the image of himself, but without his potentials and without awareness. And, to extrapolate, it is this very issue, the possibilities available to the terminally ill and suffering patient who remains conscious and competent, which voluntary euthanasia increasingly raises for resolution. For the inheritance of successful acute care is of chronic care and, for many, ultimate and often intolerable pain.

We are in trouble with definitions. For it is not obvious when death occurs. The law lords considered whether to be brain dead is to be really dead. If not, what protections are to be offered and why? Is it a greater protection to be allowed to die with dignity, or to be indefinitely maintained comatose or vegetative? It seemed as if in this debate about the mind-body problem (and about that elusive sylph, consciousness) incoherent concepts of life and death were being used. Singer, as usual, is disturbingly clear about the unsatisfactory state of our concepts and language. He says: 'Dead people are not in a coma, they are dead, and nothing can be a burden to them any more.'[16]

These are not philosophic abstractions. Ethics is for endeavour. These are excruciating and personal provocations. Many people responsibly feel that they are a burden on themselves and wish to be allowed (or helped) to die. The medical profession maintains the huge power of alone determining when death has occurred and indeed influences it in diverse ways. Judgement on when death has occurred is increasingly an *ethical* judgement, a choice about a process. Nor is death 'a moment'. It is better understood as a succession of events. It is one, too, in which doctors and other professionals make both open and concealed quality judgements.

Many ordinary people believe that they should be enabled to make informed decisions about what they want, about what control they prefer over their own bodies, about how they value their own lives and about how they would prefer to be a participant in the inevitable process of their own death. This tendency for change embraces selective non-treatment as well as active measures. The importance of the Tony Bland case resides in part in its judgement that the *possibilities* open for the individual (though not consciously, of course, in his case) are a major factor in such personal decisions.

There is, too, another important issue, another complication. This is the call for transplanted organs. For it is only when an individual is certified dead by doctors that organs can be removed for transplantation. Strict procedures are in place. However, it is only when an individual is certified dead but where there is continuing cardiac function – the heart is beating, blood circulation is oxygenating the body – that these major bodily organs are preserved in such a condition that makes it possible for them to be removed for transplantation into another living human body. Thus, as Teresa Iglesias puts it:

> the development of transplants is regarded as a practice fulfilling the aims of medicine, and consequently in accordance with its most fundamental medico-ethical principles. For in transplantation procedures the doctor seeks to benefit an individual human being, who is ill (a patient), whose life can be preserved, or his or her human condition improved, by giving him or her an organ removed from another, without harming or causing injury to that other human being (the donor) because he or she is dead. It is

clear then that to understand *when a human being is dead*, even if cardiac and respiratory functions are maintained technologically, is of great importance, particularly within the context of that branch of medicine concerned with transplants.

Yet if the individual donor were really totally, stone-cold dead (like the famous ironmongery, the door-nail, with which Dickens opens his *A Christmas Carol*) the organs would by then be useless for transplantation.[17]

The discourses concerning Tony Bland and Nancy Cruzan were several. It was variously argued that Tony Bland and Nancy Cruzan were a burden on the community, the family and the hospital. And, too, that they represented a wasted opportunity for transplants which would release others from terminal burdens. The law in Britain has accepted that Tony Bland was a loved one effectively gone for ever – unable ever to recover consciousness. However, under the law prior to this judgement he was not 'really dead', although the loss of the higher brain had severed the 'individual' from consciousness, personality, feeling, hopes, dreams and judgements. Intensive care medicine continued to regulate the body, thus embodying the integrative role of the disabled brain. Those left behind were in a personal situation of grief equally unresolved. They were denied the solace and comfort of knowing that their loved ones were beyond pain and that as much dignity and respect as possible was shown to them. The rituals of death, burial, mourning, memorial and wake were denied them. The irreversible change that death represents was, in a sense (and in a senseless sense?) in suspense. The question was, to what purpose?

Such a query applies, too, to those other patients who are apparently irreversibly comatose, yet are not diagnosed as in a persistent vegetative state (since blood continues to flow to the cortex). It is a question, too, which many *conscious* patients in intolerable pain put to themselves, to doctors and nurses and to their families and carers. This is the essential ethical judgement about the relevant ethical singularities: the capacity for the expression of self and personality, for human interaction, for enjoyable experiences, for expressing a preference about one's own quality of life and for dignity. In Tony Bland's case, none of this was within his reach despite some brain-stem functions continuing which enabled him to 'live' technologically. In a wider cast of the net, in the case of conscious and autonomous individuals, they and we have to decide which choices to allow and support. We have to decide who can best make choices about whether a life is of benefit to the person living it. And who bears the responsibility for denial. How is self-reflection and self-responsibility to be structured? The tightly regulated processes then follow.

The result of the Tony Bland case echoes far beyond the plight of the persistently vegetative patient. In the Tony Bland case the judges held that when a patient is incapable of consenting to medical treatment doctors were and are under no legal duty to continue treatment that is of no benefit to the patient. This is the view that merely to be biologically alive, but with absolutely no prospect of consciousness or awareness, is not of benefit to the patient. As others have noticed, this decision changed the rules in two crucial respects. First, the decision allowed consideration of the *quality* of life to be part of a decision as to whether a patient's life should be prolonged. Second, the judges ruled that it is lawful to pursue a course which has as its object the death of an innocent human being, which was the case with Tony Bland. Singer says: 'it is no exaggeration to say that the Bland case marks the moment at which the British courts ceased to give effect to the traditional principal of the sanctity of human life'. And: 'British law abandoned the idea that life itself is a benefit to the person living it, irrespective of its quality'.[18]

Thomas Nagel, in 1979, expressed this case in its essential:

> The value of life and its contents does not attach to mere organic survival: almost everyone would be indifferent (other things equal) between immediate death and immediate coma followed by death twenty years later without reawakening.[19]

The implication that the key to making judgements about life and death issues is the quality of a human life has a long reach. It suggests that this should be the basis for each of us to be empowered in our own decision-making about the positive and negative qualities, redeeming and intolerable qualities, burdens and benefits of our own lived-only-once lives. The sanctity of life matters a great deal and there must be a presumption to protect it. Nothingness (so far as we know) is the ultimate fate of all physical systems. Yet, since forever is a long time, it certainly seems dreadful to choose to project oneself into unimaginable (because non-existent) infinite nothingness by choice, even if none of us have any eventual option. It is a personal judgement as to whether or not how one dies does integrate and give coherence to how one lives.

There are, it seems, circumstances when the sanctity of life (and of individuals choosing to end their own lives) must be weighed against other considerations. If so (which absolutists deny), who is to do the weighing? In the case of Tony Bland, it was the doctors and the families in the framework of court direction. But for those who are competent (or who were so and made a written request), for those whose own assessment is that their prospects are merely of pointless persistence, I believe we should enable the individual to decide. For the reality of the relief of intolerable pain and the wish of the individual to guide their own death with dignity and controls, itself emphasizes the sanctity of life. How one dies matters. We do, too, see around us other nations taking serious steps, after serious thought. For example,

Dutch experience is that active euthanasia remains prohibited by law, yet is protected by both lower and supreme court decisions. It is effectively tolerated legally. Guidelines have been established which enable a voluntary decision by the patient on what to them is intolerable suffering.

Oregon and the Northern Territory of Australia have new policy approaches to these moral questions. The change in the law in Oregon following the referendum in November 1994, and the new *Rights of the Terminally Ill Act* in the Northern Territory of Australia, suggest that changes can be made which cumulate public support. These seem to be both workable and responsibly undertaken by all concerned. But it is still true that we remain intolerant of even responsible expressions of such ideas. This itself reflects the anxiety that what we have here is a 'slippery slope'. Even so, in my estimate, there seems likely to be a gradual but global change in our ethics, as more people, faced with terrible pain which can no longer be alleviated, ask 'Doctor, do I have a choice?', and 'Why not?' One medical response is to withhold treatment, which many clearly agree to do. But this can allow much of the suffering to remain, even if partially alleviated by drugs. Thus, many argue for active euthanasia once the initial decision not to prolong the agony has been made. They argue, too, that there is no moral difference between active and passive euthanasia. Nor must there inevitably be a slippery slope. This is clearly a judgement which many find difficult to endorse – and this despite the perception that once passive euthanasia has been accepted this has already put in place the idea that in a particular instance death is no greater an evil than the patient's continued painful existence. As James Rachels noted:

> To say otherwise is to endorse the option that leads to more suffering rather than less, and is contrary to the humanitarian impulse that prompts the decision not to prolong his life in the first place.[20]

Balance

It is always about balance and interpretation. The religious commentator, *qua* adventure novelist, Daniel Defoe, says in *Robinson Crusoe* that: 'All evils are to be considered with the good that is in them, and with what worse attends them'. And further:

> Upon the whole, here was an undoubted testimony, that there was scarce any condition in the world so miserable, but there was something negative or something positive to be thankful for in it; and let this stand as a direction from the experience of the most miserable of all conditions in this world, that we may always find

in it something to comfort our selves from, and to set in the description of good and evil, on the credit side of the accompt.[21]

This view celebrates life, as Dworkin has shown. These, however, remain potentially criminal matters. If society changes its view it must change the law as it relates to the legal consequences for doctors. This has been done tacitly in Holland and more directly in the Northern Territory of Australia.

In Britain, the implications of the judgement in the Tony Bland case are commodious. They have extensive implications for possible changes in the laws concerning voluntary and non-voluntary euthanasia – about how we regulate ending life by actively doing something and how we regulate ending life by doing nothing. That is, what doctors do or may do intentionally to kill a patient or to intentionally allow a patient to die. We already know that in practice these can be very fine, even invisible, distinctions. The basis of judgements about quality of life and how individual choices can be legally expressed and protected is (as Singer has, in my view, rightly argued) the potential basis of a new and workable ethics. We need one which can help construct good law which itself can bear ethical weight. What Dworkin says is also a fundamental reference, for we do die in the shadow of our whole lives.

Meanwhile, we sustain difficulties in practice as we seek to maintain fine distinctions. The British law lord, Lord Browne-Wilkinson, has said here:

> How can it be lawful to allow a patient to die slowly, though painlessly, over a period of weeks from lack of food but unlawful to produce his immediate death by a lethal injection, thereby saving his family from yet another ordeal to add to the tragedy that has already struck them? I find it difficult to find a moral answer to that question.[22]

Yet British law seeks to maintain that distinction, between acts of omission and the act of commission or 'mercy killing'. The daily reality is that the distinction between a positive and a negative act is difficult to determine. It seems to have little coherent ethical basis. It may, indeed, have less impact on actualite than has been thought.

A special problem posed by the Tony Bland case was that of substituted judgements – that is, what would the disabled individual have wanted, if he had been able to express himself? Here, again, the emphasis should be not merely on the body but on the uniqueness of the individual personality, of the conscious *person*. For the issue is whether or not the persistence of the body is what we mean – or rather, what the individual concerned may mean – by 'life'. Increasingly – and this is one lesson from the case of the young widow who wished to receive the stored sperm of her dead husband – people may wish to specify in writing what they would want in as many specific circumstances as they can envisage. Otherwise, it is difficult for the 'proxy' ever conclusively to answer such questions as what someone would want or would have wanted. Children and fetuses, of course, pose special problems of the expression and interpretation of 'their interests' since these cannot necessarily be 'known' at all.

Singer puts these issues with his exemplary lucidity and sensitivity:

> The advances of medical technology have forced us to think about issues that we previously had no need to face. When there was nothing we could do to preserve the lives of fetuses inside the bodies of pregnant women whose brains had died, we did not have to make up our minds about the status of a fetus whose mother had died months before it could be born. When infants without brains never lived more than a few days, and organ transplantation did not exist, it was easy enough to say that *every* human being has a right to life. We did not have to ask whether some lives are more valuable than others. Now we cannot avoid that question, unless we are willing to be propelled along willy-nilly by the desires of doctors and scientists to be the first with the next medical miracle. Technology creates an imperative: 'If we can do it, we will do it.' Ethics asks: 'We can do it, but should we do it?' But the ethic within which we try to answer this question stands on shaky foundations that few of us now accept. Confused and contradictory judgements are the result.[23]

We do, of course, seek to maintain commitments which prove in practice to be self-contradictory, as Berlin shows. And so perhaps we do need to be more suspicious of a law which requires heroic medical measures which can produce cases where there is more suffering than solace. This is not only (although, inevitably it is undeniably partly) an issue of resources. It is chiefly a moral and ethical question. That is, if we wish to avoid outcomes which no-one wants, and to protect people from these. The law, too, needs to maintain social consent while keeping pace with new dilemmas and new boundary definitions.

These changes in ethical and moral positions ask us to think deeply about life, death and pain. These issues ask us to think about choice, about autonomy and about incommensurable choices. They ask us what kind of society we wish to live in. They pose those dilemmas and balances to be faced or struck. We should notice, too, that the dreaded frontier is not only death. It can be, even more fearfully for many, essentially insupportable pain and indignity, the loss of choice and thus of life-definition in one's own terms.

We assume that death is necessarily bad. But philosophy has suggested that this itself may be an odd idea. Thomas Nagel, for example, discusses whether if death is the unequivocal and permanent end of our existence it is a bad thing to die. And if death is itself an evil, how great an evil and of what kind. As Nagel points out (one may think unsurprisingly), 'there is conspicuous disagreement about the matter'. Nagel asks whether anything can be bad for a man without being positively unpleasant for him. And since death is to be nothing then there can be no experience of unpleasantness since no experiences are possible once one is dead. It is an awful choice, between pain and nothingness, between suffering in an ever and nothingness in a forever. But people show courage in facing it. Nagel says, however, that:

> there are special difficulties, in the case of death, about how the supposed misfortune is to be assigned to a subject at all. There is doubt both as to *who* its subject is, and as to *when* he undergoes it. So long as a person exists, he has not yet died, and once he has died, he no longer exists; so there seems to be no time when death, if it is a misfortune, can be ascribed to its unfortunate subject.[24]

This is to me logically clear, but intuitively disagreeable, as is the argument that death is merely the mirror image of the abyss prior to one's own birth. For death is the loss of the familiar outline of the future. It was this loss which we ascribed to Tony Bland and which was in good part his tragedy. For, in the precise language of the ethicist, death 'is an abrupt cancellation of indefinitely extensive possible goods'.[25] The tragedy of Tony Bland is especially harsh if we believe that life is all we have – itself, grounds for disputation – and the loss of life the greatest loss we can sustain. But Nagel observes:

> On the other hand it may be objected that death deprives this supposed loss of its subject, and that if we realise that death is not an unimaginable condition of the persisting person, but a mere blank, we will see that it can have no value whatever, positive or negative.[26]

Is this to say, do not be concerned for whom the bell tolls, for it tolls for nobody? It is, too, curiously discomforting to consider Francis Bacon's words that 'no man knows his own death'. For even if death is not logically experienced at all, our individual loss is of the unlived life we feel entitled to. We know that death entails this loss, however old we survive to be. And the challenge to the conscious person in pain is that there is a loss no matter how much life has been lived. We generally think it is good to be alive, and not good to be dead. It takes courage to ask for death and to wish to control the circumstances, even if this rounds out a life.

Nagel tells us that death has no positive features (so far as we know). Its features are negative, since it brings to an end all of life's goods, including its difficulties and dilemmas. As he says: 'if death is an evil, it is the *loss of life*, rather than the state of being dead, or non-existent, or unconscious, that is objectionable'. And: 'It is sometimes suggested that what we really mind is the process of *dying*. But I should not really object to dying if it were not followed by death'.[27] It is a relative judgement for the individual whether suffering is preferable to non-existence. Tony Bland did not have a choice. But since death for us all is ultimately unavoidable, one can see that people may wish to balance the loss of life (for example, from a cancer with its terminal pain and suffering) against the knowledge that death removes all knowledge but also all pain. For each of us the deprivation and loss remains tragic. Its facilitation in some circumstances, as in Holland and now in a part of Australia, seems likely to encourage a global wish for choice. If so, this must be the subject of the utmost kindness and supportiveness within the law. As Shakespeare says, this may:

> ease them of their griefs, Their fears of hostile strokes, their Aches losses, Their pangs of love, with other incident throwes, That Natures fragile Vessel doth sustaine in life's uncertain voyage.[28]

A great philosopher, David Hume, of course addressed these issues in his classic commentary on suicide. This is apposite to those conscious and autonomous, informed and advised patients asking for death. They do so on the basis of personal moral beliefs. It is, too, a social and moral question as to whether anyone has the right to decide how much pain and suffering another should have to endure if there are alternatives which they seek. It is a similar question as to whether or not society should expect an individual to tolerate losing the dignity and ability to eat, walk, move, speak, swallow and exercise self-control without assistance and pain. A difficulty is that suicide has been de-criminalized. Yet people who wish for death as a release from what is to them an unbearable situation which will not improve or be relieved in any other way, often decide such a wish when it is beyond their own capacity to achieve it for themselves.

Clearly, a policy of voluntary euthanasia requires on one side a re-definition of good medical practice. On the other side of the argument is the requirement to protect the lives of the vulnerable. As Hume wrote: 'The contest is here more equal between the distemper and the medicine'.[29] Yet he was himself an advocate:

> 'I go out of life, and put a period to a being, which, were it to continue, would render me miserable ... I am only convinced of a matter of fact ... that human life may be unhappy, and that my existence, if further prolonged, would become ineligible: but I thank providence, both for the good which I have already

enjoyed, and for the power with which I am endc
the ill that threatens me ... when the horror of pa
the love of life; when a voluntary action anticipati
blind causes ... That suicide may often be consister.
and with our duty to ourselves, no one can questioi
that age, sickness, or misfortune may render life a
make it worse even than annihilation ... I believe t ___.o man
ever threw away life, while it was worth keeping ... For such is
our natural horror of death, that small motives will never be able
to reconcile us to it.[30]

Singer summarizes a number of key points which make clear the nature of
these debates. Thus:

> The desire for control over how we die marks a sharp turning
> away from the sanctity of life ethic. It will not be satisfied by the
> concessions to patient autonomy within the framework of that
> ethic – a right to refuse 'extraordinary means' of medical treat-
> ment, or to employ drugs like morphine that are intended to relieve
> pain, but have the unintended but foreseen side-effect of short-
> ening life. The right to refuse medical treatment can help only
> in the limited number of cases in which it leads to a swift and
> painless death. Most cancer patients, for instance, are not in this
> situation. They are more likely to be helped by liberal injections
> of morphine.[31]

However, for those who wish to choose their own time of dying, with their
family around them, this is not a sufficient solution. Nor will it, I think,
be a sustainable compromise. For the Dutch, Oregon and Australian experiences will influence what happens elsewhere in an increasingly mono-
cultural world.[32]

> I think that the free exercise of choice in autonomy will involve many more
> of us in a medical decision to end a life if its quality has deteriorated to an un-
> acceptable point. Only we can decide this for ourselves. We cannot control
> how we are born. But many will wish to control how they die. We speak of
> an idea whose time has come; this is a time whose idea has come. Especially
> so if we are to be able to respond to Shakespeare's call, 'to give healthful
> welcome to their shipwrack'd'.[33] And to take seriously the Japanese experi-
> ence and the significance of self-esteem and thus empowerment as a trigger
> for good health. For, as Sterne says in the dedication to *Tristram Shandy*:

> > I live in a constant endeavour to fence against the infirmities of
> > ill health, and other evils of life, by mirth; being firmly persuaded
> > that every time a man smiles, but much more so, when he laughs,
> > it adds something to this Fragment of Life.[34]

e is clearly pressure for choice about choice. There are persuasive advo-
ates that we should re-set our moral chronometers by the regular rhythm
of autonomy – like the ball that drops down the weather vane mast in the
Meridian Courtyard at Greenwich every day, 'like the fireman descending a
very short pole'.[35] We require a new ethics and new law which meets these
imperatives, if, in Francis Bacon's words, we are to stand 'upon the vantage
ground of truth'. This is always an elusive and never an easy task. Hamlet
could not locate it securely. The meaning of the ghost in the Danish play
remains a puzzle. And, as Bacon famously wrote: 'What is truth, said jesting
Pilate, and would not stay for an answer'.[36]

Notes

1   See Hardy H (ed.) (1996) *Isaiah Berlin. The sense of reality: studies in
    ideas and their history.* Chatto & Windus, London, p. 5.

2   Shakespeare, *All's Well That Ends Well*, Act 2, scene 1.

3   See Page N (ed.) (1971) *Charles Dickens: Bleak House.* Penguin
    English Library, London, p. 684.

4   See Andre J (1992) Learning to see: moral growth during medical
    training. *J. Med. Ethics* **18**: 148–52. Also see Entwhistle V, Watt IS and
    Herring JE (1996) *An introduction for consumer health information
    providers.* King's Fund, London – a missed opportunity in a document
    otherwise having potential for influencing real actions for isolating
    why problems arise and how they could be managed for change. It is
    interesting to note how often an attempt from within the system is
    itself a symptom, not a solution.

5   For an extensive analysis concerning empowerment, politicians and
    power see my *'Only a novel!' Jane Austen, hypertext and the story of
    patient power.* In: Marshall M (ed.) (1996) *Sense and sensibility in
    health care.* BMJ Publishing, London. See also my *'Virtual Reality
    Health Councils' in tomorrow's high streets.* In: *Health Service Journal*
    106(5527): 2 (Rhône-Poulenc Rorer bound insert entitled *Three's a
    crowd*).

6   See Roszak T (1994) *The cult of information: a neo-Luddite treatise on
    high-tech, artificial intelligence and the true art of thinking.* (2nd ed.)
    University of California Press, Berkeley.

7   Page N (ed.) (1971), op.cit., p. 876.

8   See, amongst his writings, Gould SJ (1989) *Wonderful Life: The
    Burgess shale and the nature of history.* Hutchinson Radius, London.

9   See *Airedale NHS Trust v. Bland (CA)*, 19 February 1993, 2 WLR
    316–400 and *Cruzan v. Director, Missouri Department of Health*
    (1990) 110, Supreme Court, 2841. See also Dworkin R (1993) *Life's
    dominion: an argument about abortion and euthanasia*. Alfred A
    Knopf, New York and Singer P (1995) *Rethinking life and death: the
    collapse of our traditional ethics*. OUP, Oxford. Also, Keown J (1993)
    Courting euthanasia? Tony Bland and the Law Lords. *Ethics &
    Medicine* 8: 3 and Cranford RE (1988) The persistent vegetative state:
    the medical reality (getting the facts straight). *Hastings Center Report*
    18(1): 27–8.

10 See Cramb A (1996) Brother in 'mercy killing' goes free. In: *The Daily
    Telegraph*, 15 October 1996.

11 See Dyer C (1996) Widow will fight on to have baby by husband.
    In: *The Guardian*, 18 October 1996; Gibb F and Wilkins E (1996),
    Law may change as widow loses plea for baby; Wilkins E (1996) Wife
    will continue fight to have dead husband's baby; Gibb F (1996)
    Warnock blames herself for not foreseeing such a case; Gibb F (1996)
    Court powerless to override act; Law Report (*Regina v. Human
    Fertilisation and Embryology Authority, ex parte Blood*) – all in *The
    Times*, 18 October 1996; Shaw T (1996) I'll fight on to have my
    husband's baby, says widow. In: *The Daily Telegraph*, 18 October
    1996; Wilkins E and Thomson A (1996) Public rallies behind widow
    who wants baby. In: *The Times*, 19 October 1996.

12 See William Pickering, Kindness, prescribed and natural, in medi-
    cine, forthcoming in *J. Med. Ethics* February 1997. I am grateful to
    Dr Pickering for letting me read the typescript in advance of publica-
    tion. Dr Pickering stresses that we should not only focus on the com-
    plicated issues but also on ordinary everyday life and work. For
    example, in the activity of GPs the ethical imperative is to be kind and
    ethical in judging whether an individual needs a particular treatment
    and will benefit from it.

13 Dr William Pickering, private conversation, 18 October 1996.

14 See *Cruzan v. Director, Missouri Department of Health* (1990), op.cit.
    See especially the discussions in Dworkin (1993), op.cit. and Singer
    (1995), op.cit., together with the references they give.

15 See Pallis C (1983) *ABC of brain stem death*. BMJ Publications,
    London.

16 Singer (1995), op.cit., pp. 65–8.

17 See Iglesias T (1995) Ethics, brain-death and the medical concept of
    the human being. *Medico-legal Journal of Ireland* 1(2): 51–7. Also
    Dickens C (1843) *A Christmas carol*. In: Slater M (ed.) (1995) *The
    Christmas Books*. Volume 1. Classics edition. Penguin, London, p. 1.

18   See Singer (1995), op.cit., p. 149. For a full discussion of the Dutch and Oregon positions see Singer (1995), *ibid.*, and the sources he cites especially in Chapter 7, *Asking for death*. See also Singer P (1993) (2nd ed.) *Practical ethics*. CUP, Cambridge especially Chapter 7, *Taking life: humans* and his references. Saunders C (1992) Voluntary euthanasia. *Palliative Medicine* 6: 1–5 is helpful, as are her references. She queries the decision-making processes in Holland and the adequacy of palliative care. On the Northern Territory of Australia, see my discussion of *The Rights of the Terminally Ill Act 1995* in the Introduction and lecture here. Also, Christie A and Hassan R (1994) Management of death, dying and euthanasia: attitudes and practices of medical practitioners in South Australia. *J. Med. Ethics* 20: 41–6; Dworkin R (1993), op.cit.; Rachels J (1994) Active and passive euthanasia. In: Singer (1993), op.cit., p. 30. But see Hawkes N (1996) Elderly wary of mercy killing, survey shows. In: *The Times*, 23 October 1996 reporting a study in *Archives of Internal Medicine*.

19   See Nagel T (1986) Death. In: Singer P (ed.) *Applied ethics*. OUP, Oxford.

20   See Rachels J (1994), op.cit., p. 30.

21   See Ross A (ed.) (1965) *Daniel Defoe. The life and adventures of Robinson Crusoe* (1719). Penguin Books.

22   *Airedale NHS Trust v. Bland (CA)*, op.cit., p. 387.

23   Singer P (1995), op.cit., p. 19.

24   Nagel T (1986), op.cit., p. 12.

25   Nagel T (1986), *ibid.*, p. 18.

26   Nagel T (1986), *ibid.*, p. 9.

27   Nagel T (1986), *ibid.*, p. 11.

28   Shakespeare, *Timon of Athens*, Act 5, scene 1.

29   See Hume D (1986) Of suicide. In: Singer P (1986), op.cit. (Reprinted from Green TD and Gosse TH (eds) (1874–5) *The Philosophical Works of David Hume*. London.)

30   Hume D (1986), *ibid.*, pp. 23–6.

31   Singer P (1995), op.cit., p. 147.

32   See especially Dworkin R (1993), op.cit. and Singer P (1995), op.cit. for the Dutch and the American experiences including the referenda in California. On how the rationing dilemmas will be personalized by interactive multi-media technology see my essay on health care futures and new technologies where I give an account of how people will confer internationally on health care issues, drawing on the narrative

experiences of others – see *'Only a novel!' Jane Austen, hypertext and the story of patient power*, op.cit. It is no surprise that the computer software used in the Northern Territory of Australia to permit voluntary euthanasia is now being made available on the Internet. See Maynard R (1996) 'Mercy killing' kit to go on Internet. In: *The Times*, 16 October 1996.

33 Shakespeare, *The Comedy of Errors*, Act 1, scene 1.

34 See Laurence Sterne's, *Tristram Shandy*. The dedication first appeared in Volumes i and ii of the second edition in April 1760.

35 See Sobel D (1996) *Longitude: the true story of a lone genius who solved the greatest scientific problem of his time*. Fourth Estate, London, pp. 168–9.

36 See *Francis Bacon: the essays* (1625). Edited Penguin edition, p. 1.

Index